T0144427

BASIC HEALTH PUBLICATIONS USER'S GUIDE

TO ANTIOXIDANT SUPPLEMENTS

Discover How Natural Antioxidants Can Reduce Your Risk of Heart Disease, Cancer, and Alzheimer's Disease.

JACK CHALLEM AND
MELISSA BLOCK
JACK CHALLEM Series Editor

The information contained in this book is based upon the research and personal and professional experiences of the authors. It is not intended as a substitute for consulting with your physician or other healthcare provider. Any attempt to diagnose and treat an illness should be done under the direction of a healthcare professional. The publisher does not advocate the use of any particular healthcare protocol but believes the information in this book should be available to the public. The publisher and authors are not responsible for any adverse effects or consequences resulting from the use of the suggestions, preparations, or procedures discussed in this book. Should the reader have any questions concerning the appropriateness of any procedures or preparations mentioned, the authors and the publisher strongly suggest consulting a professional healthcare advisor.

Series Editor: Jack Challem
Editor: Tara Durkin
Typesetter: Gary A. Rosenberg
Series Cover Designer: Mike Stromberg

Basic Health Publications User's Guides are published by Basic Health Publications, Inc.

CONTENTS

INTRODUCTION

If you could take a pill each day that would most likely lengthen your life span while significantly reducing your chances of ending up with occlusive heart disease, heart failure, cancer, stroke, Alzheimer's disease, complications from diabetes, eye diseases causing blindness, rheumatoid arthritis, TMJ (temporomandibular joint) disorder, skin diseases, and muscle soreness following exercise, would you take it?

There's no drug that will do all that, you might be thinking. *That's impossible! If there were, every doctor would have every patient on it.* True. No *drug* can do this. But bear with us. Would you take such a pill if it existed?

What's the catch? you may wonder. *Will there be scary side effects?* No. *Is it outrageously expensive?* No: at most, a few dollars a day; at least, a few pennies a day. *Is it something that has been barely researched—something that no one really knows the risks and benefits of?* No, this substance has been rigorously studied since the middle of the twentieth century. *Will I have to trade my first-born child?* Okay, now you're being silly. Let's have an answer: Would you take the substance or not?

Well, yes, of course!

So would we. What is this miraculous pill to which we are referring? It—or, more accurately, *they*—are the subject of this book, and of extensive research in laboratories and medical centers all over the world. We are talking about antioxidants.

It all goes back to a research chemist named Denham Harman, who in November 1954 had a "eureka!" moment. Dr. Harman thought he had figured out what drives the aging process.

In December of 1945, his wife had showed him an article about the work of Russian researchers who were attempting to extend the human life span, and it had intrigued him. Finally, sitting at his desk nine years later, it came to him: *the cause of aging is oxidation.*

His past work for the Shell Oil Company had involved free-radical chemistry, but at that time, no one had an inkling that there would ever be a connection drawn between free radicals and aging. No scientist had ever detected free-radical activity in human cells.

Once Dr. Harman had his "eureka" moment, he set about trying to find free radicals in living systems. This did not prove to be an easy task, but by the 1960s—with the help of many other scientists who came to see the brilliance of what he was doing—studies had established that free radicals were indeed a product of cellular metabolism (more on this later) and that supplementation with antioxidant substances reliably increased the life expectancy of lab animals.

At this writing, Dr. Harman is still hard at work. He is in his late eighties, yet he continues to rise at 4:30 each morning to go to his office at the University of Nebraska, Omaha, where he is professor emeritus. He sits at his desk for eight to nine hours a day, poring over scientific research and working on new research strategies that will—he hopes—permanently move antioxidant supplementation into the mainstream of modern life.

Dr. Harman's lonely early research sowed the seeds for the current explosion of antioxidant research. There are more than 111,000 scientific studies, published in peer-reviewed scientific journals, that concern antioxidants and their activity in animal and human cells. No theory about chronic or age-related disease can last long without considering the role free radicals play in their onset and progression.

In these pages, you will learn exactly what a free radical is, and why it is harmful. You'll see the connection between free radicals and diabetes, heart disease, cancer, and Alzheimer's disease. And you'll find out that a lot of the agents that help us resist the onslaught of free radicals—the antioxidants—may well be our best protection against these diseases.

In Chapter 1, we'll go into greater detail about the science of free radicals and antioxidants—just enough to give you a complete understanding of the chapters that follow. Have a pencil handy when you get to Chapter 2 because we're going to establish just how much you need supplemental antioxidants with a not-too-scientific quiz. Chapters 3, 4, 5, and 6 will get to the nitty-gritty, describing the research that has demonstrated the benefits of antioxidant vitamins and minerals; of *endogenous* (made in the body) antioxidants that work even greater magic when taken as supplements; and of antioxidants found in herbs and other plants, edible and not. Finally, in the Conclusion, we'll help you see how to apply all the science to your life and your health.

Some of these nutrients will be familiar to you; some, you may already be using. Others will be totally new. We won't mention anything in these pages that has not been thoroughly researched. Once you've finished reading this book, we're sure that you will be convinced that antioxidant nutrients are an indispensable part of a healthy lifestyle—and that they can be used to prevent, and to help the body heal from, some of the most common health problems that threaten us from middle age onward.

CHAPTER 1

FREE RADICALS AND ANTIOXIDANTS DEMYSTIFIED

You've probably heard a lot of talk about free radicals and antioxidants. You may have made some attempt to figure out just what exactly they are, and you may even have tried to learn which antioxidants you should take to protect and promote good health. This book will take you to the next level: it will apprise you of what is currently understood about antioxidants, and it will help you decide which ones you ought to be taking.

Antioxidants are not drugs, although some drugs can have an antioxidant effect in the body. And although many researchers are currently transforming some natural antioxidants into drugs, the best antioxidants come directly from nature. Some come from foods; some come from plants that are not eaten as food; still others are made within the living cells of the body, and have been isolated and studied as nutritional supplements.

Simply put, antioxidants neutralize free radicals. Free radicals are atoms or atomic groups that contain unpaired electrons.

A Closer Look At Free Radicals

Think back to your high-school chemistry class. Remember that atoms are the stuff from which molecules are made; they are the smallest component of matter. See if you can visualize that plastic model your teacher pulled out to illustrate her description of an atom. There's the nucleus, represented as a central sphere, half positively charged protons and half neutrally charged neutrons. Around the nucleus, electrons travel in an orbiting pathway. (Any modern chemist or physicist will tell you that this model is extremely simplistic, but it suits our purposes just fine.)

Like many people, electrons prefer to exist in a paired state. When an electron is removed from its pair, the remaining electron will indiscriminately pick up electrons from other atoms. (Again, the behaviors of human couples come to mind.) Electrons can be stolen from fats, proteins—even DNA, the genetic material that dictates the activity of every cell. This sets up a chain reaction that can cause substantial biological damage.

Oxidation
The loss of one of a pair of electrons.

Reduction
The gaining of an electron to complete a pair.

The loss of one of a pair of electrons is known as *oxidation*. When an electron is added back to complete the electron pairing, that's *reduction* in action. Within virtually every cell of the bodies of animals and humans, a constant cycle of oxidation and reduction is taking place.

Antioxidants Save the Day

The body employs antioxidants to *reduce* free radicals and prevent the damage that they can do. Antioxidants donate electrons to free radicals, halting the chain reaction and stabilizing the atom that has been tearing around trying to find a match for its lovelorn unpaired electron.

Research in this field has established, beyond a doubt, that an overabundance of free radicals relative to antioxidants plays a substantial role in the development of age-related diseases and in the aging process. In other words, when there are more free radicals than the body's antioxidants can handle, we grow old faster, and we get sicker in the process.

Fortunately, there is a lot you can do to improve your body's capacity for "quenching" free radicals.

With an intelligent, moderate, and well-balanced program of antioxidant nutrient supplementation, you can demonstrably raise the concentration of antioxidant substances in your bloodstream and within the cells of your body.

Free Radicals and Oxidation: An Even Closer Look

Your body contains several organ systems that each do their own part to keep you alive and thriving. The cells that make up those organs, it turns out, have their own organs, which scientists call *organelles*. Within each of the 60 trillion cells of your body are microscopic organelles called *mitochondria*. The mitochondria are the "power plants" of cells; they are responsible for transforming fuel (carbohydrates and fats) into energy. They provide the energy necessary to make heart cells beat, lung cells breathe, liver cells filter the blood and eliminate toxins, and brain cells think.

Within each mitochondrion, dozens of chemical reactions convert carbohydrates and fats to the chemical currency of energy: *adenosine triphosphate*, or ATP. These chemical reactions—collectively known as the *Krebs cycle* and *oxidative phosphorylation*—require the participation of many vitamins, minerals, and antioxidants.

In the process of creating ATP (which is then partially broken down to release chemical energy wherever it is needed), mitochondria become ground zero for the production of free radicals. Free radicals are a natural byproduct of metabolism, and they are necessary to sustain the metabolic process. Unfortunately, they also cause damage to proteins, fats, and DNA (deoxyribonucleic acid), the biological code that programs our cells.

In trying to become a part of an intact molecule, this fragment of a molecule—which is, in essence, what a free radical is—modifies and possibly permanently damages the molecule it is trying to become a part of. As we age, the body's ability to prevent and repair this damage declines, and this is the root of the characteristic changes and maladies that arise as we grow older.

Free-Radical Damage to Proteins

While most of us think of protein as something we get from foods, the truth is that all living things are built from proteins. A protein is a large molecule composed of one or more chains of amino acids in a specific order. The order of the amino acids in each protein is determined by genetic information encoded in the DNA of each cell.

Proteins are required for the structure, function, and regulation of the body's cells, tissues, and organs. Hormones, enzymes, and antibodies are all proteins. Free-radical attack can lead to structural changes in proteins, which, in turn, hampers their ability to do their jobs in the body.

Oxidative damage to proteins has been implicated as a cause of Alzheimer's disease. Free-radical reactions with proteins and fats in the skin are a major cause of the external aging process.

Free-Radical Damage to Fats

The membranes of all cells and the sheaths that surround nerve cells are composed of fats. The brain is 60 percent fat. Fats—especially polyunsaturated fats, the kind that are most prevalent in the body—are highly vulnerable to oxidative attack. Wastes and fuel don't pass through cell membranes as easily once the membrane's fats have been oxidized. In the end, accumulated damage from membrane oxidation makes a significant contribution to aging throughout the body.

Millions of Americans have high cholesterol. What this usually means is that there are high levels of *low-density lipoproteins,* or *LDL,* and low levels of *high-density lipoproteins,* or *HDL.* It was once believed that simply having high LDL relative to HDL was an important cause of cardiovascular disease, but new evidence has all but proven that *oxidative modification* of LDL—that is, free-radical attack that triggers alterations in LDL—is the key to making this "bad" type of cholesterol truly *atherogenic* (harmful to artery walls).

LDL isn't all bad. It carries fat-soluble nutrients such as vitamin E and beta-carotene through the blood. When we don't consume enough antioxidant nutrients, however, LDL can become oxidized by a buildup of free radicals. Oxidative modification, which results from this buildup, causes the immune system to react against LDL; normally, LDL causes no immune reaction. White blood cells are dispatched to engulf the LDL as though it were bacteria. Then, *adhesion molecules* are released from the surface of the LDL-engorged white blood cells and become stuck to artery walls. Other inflammatory substances, such as *C-reactive protein* (CRP) and *interleukin-6* (IL-6) are drawn into the fray, and the end result is a swollen, inflamed plaque that may obstruct the flow of blood through the artery. This all begins with a lack of antioxidant nutrients.

Free-Radical Damage to DNA

DNA contains biological instructions for cells that tell them how to grow, change, and perform their everyday functions. Nearly every one of our 60 trillion cells contains a complete set of these instructions, and select aspects of those instructions are activated within different types of cells.

When free radicals attack DNA, they can garble, or *mutate*, these instructions in ways that cause cells to become cancerous. They become *undifferentiated*, meaning that they lose the characteristics that allow them to perform special functions. For example: a cancerous liver cell can't cleanse the blood of toxins; a cancerous lung cell can't move oxygen in and out of the bloodstream.

Cells that have become cancerous also multiply far more rapidly than healthy cells. They are immortal—as long as they have fuel and a place to grow, they do not die. (Healthy cells, on the other hand, are programmed to die and to be replaced by new cells periodically; this programmed cell death is called *apoptosis*.) Cancer cells use up energy and take up space needed by the organ to do its job. Once cancerous cells have multiplied enough to become a tumor, they often spread to other parts of the body through the lymph vessels. Eventually, cancerous cells can overwhelm the function of organ systems and cause death.

Antioxidants have been found to prevent oxidative modification of DNA, which initiates cancer. They may also help to slow cancer's progression, assisting the body in mounting defenses that stop or reverse its growth.

If Antioxidants Are So Great, Why Don't Doctors Prescribe Them?

If the scientific evidence in favor of antioxidant supplementation is as strong as we are suggesting, why hasn't it been wholeheartedly embraced by the medical establishment? The answer to this question has more to do with politics and money than it has to do with science. Natural substances receive little attention from the medical community because they are not profitable products for pharmaceutical companies.

Nearly all drugs are created from molecules that are not found in nature. Sometimes they are made from natural substances that have been "tweaked" to make them unnatural; sometimes they are built from scratch. These unnatural molecules tend to have more dramatic effects on the body than natural molecules. (This is why drugs are more dangerous than natural molecules, causing upwards of 100,000 deaths and millions of adverse events every year.)

Their unnaturalness is exactly what makes it possible for them to become patented. Drug companies make the most profit when they patent their products, because it means they don't have to compete with others who are making the same thing. They can charge what they like. The pharmaceutical industry has grown extremely rich based on modern drug-patenting regulations. In turn, drug companies use their riches to fund research on their newest products, and to "educate" doctors and consumers about the value of those products. Drug companies also strongly influence government-run health education programs, which strive to give the impression that the only way to deal with disease is through the use of powerful pharmaceutical agents. The value of natural antioxidant supplements for the protection and promotion of health isn't even on the radar of drug companies, healthcare administrators, or the majority of physicians.

Natural antioxidants like those described in this book are not patentable (with the exception of a few that have special delivery systems or special combinations or permutations of natural substances; for example, Pycnogenol is a patented extract from maritime pine tree bark, and certain forms of coenzyme Q_{10} are patented because they are made in an oil base designed to improve absorption). This is one reason why you haven't heard more about natural antioxidants, despite the fact that their beneficial effects on health have been firmly established with scientific studies every bit as rigorous (and sometimes far more so!) than those used to establish the safety and efficacy of prescription drugs.

Another reason why antioxidants are not widely recommended by medical doctors is because Western medicine is less a healthcare system than a disease-care system. The focus is on fixing people who are broken rather than fortifying the

body so that it can defend itself against disease—
and so that it can heal itself if disease does strike.

Antioxidants Are Not "Magic Bullets"

Antioxidant supplementation is an excellent support for good health, but it does not cure disease. It helps the body maintain its own defenses against disease, and when disease strikes, antioxidants can promote healing, but it's not a matter of "take this pill and your disease will go away."

We have been led to expect "magic bullet" treatments, instantaneous cures for illness that allow us not only to get better right away but also to let us get on with our busy lives even when we are sick. Antibiotics and painkillers can accomplish these ends. Increasingly, however, chronic conditions such as heart disease, cancer, and Alzheimer's disease are baffling the mainstream medical model. There is no cure for these diseases; there are drugs and surgeries to try to buy us time, to slow their progression, but no cure.

Antioxidant supplementation works best when it is used consistently and preventatively—to support optimal health at the level of every cell, every protein, every fat molecule, each spiral of DNA.

This is not to say that antioxidant supplements are useless in the face of illness. On the contrary: antioxidants in higher dosages can do a lot for you when you become sick. It's important, however, to achieve a good balance of antioxidant nutrients, and to use the forms that research has demonstrated work best.

CHAPTER 2

WHAT'S YOUR OXIDATION SCORE?

Got your pencil? Let's see how you do on this questionnaire, which we have designed to help you figure out which antioxidants you could benefit from, and the dosage ranges that are likely to suit your individual needs.

Each question has up to five possible answers. Each response corresponds to a certain number of points, as listed. Write the point count for each question in the far-right margin, then add the points up once you've completed the questionnaire.

1. How many servings of vegetables and fruit do you eat each day? (A serving consists of one medium-sized fruit; $1/2$ cup raw, cooked, or canned fruits or vegetables; or 1 cup of salad greens.)
   Vegetables and fruits are the best natural sources of antioxidant nutrition.
   a) 5 per day or more—1 point
   b) 4 per day—2 points
   c) 3 per day—3 points
   d) 2 per day—4 points
   e) 1 per day or fewer—5 points

2. Do you use a lot of herbs and spices in your cooking—particularly, garlic, onion, curry, rosemary, sage, cayenne, turmeric? Score yourself according to the number of times per day you eat one or more of these herbs and spices.

Herbs and spices are loaded with antioxidant substances—many of which are under intense study for their use as disease preventatives and therapies, and have been used by traditional medical practices for centuries.

a) 5 times or more—1

b) 4 times—2

c) 3 times—3

d) 2 times—4

e) 1 time or less—5

3. How many hours a week do you spend trying to tan your skin in the sun or in a tanning booth? *Direct exposure to UV radiation breeds lots of free radicals in the skin. Sunscreen may help prevent burns, but there is no proof that it prevents free-radical formation.*

a) 1 hour or less—1

b) 2 hours—2

c) 3 hours—3

d) 4 hours—4

e) 5 hours or more—5

4. Do you smoke? (If you are exposed to secondary smoke, give yourself 2 or 3 points.) *Cigarette smoke is one of the most pernicious sources of free radicals. Smokeless tobacco has this effect as well.*

a) no, I don't smoke at all—1

b) I am around smoke occasionally—2

c) I am around smoke often—3

d) I smoke less than ten cigarettes a day—4

e) I smoke more than ten cigarettes a day—5

5. How many alcoholic drinks do you have per week? (Don't count red wine, unless you drink more than a glass a day.)

Drinking too much beer or hard liquor has been found to increase the risk of oral cancers, and this may be partly due to free-radical stress in the mouth and throat.

a) 1 drink or fewer—1

b) 2 drinks—2

c) 3 drinks—3

d) 4 drinks—4

e) 5 drinks or more—5

6. How hard do you exercise? (If you don't exercise at all, choose d.)

Moderate exercise improves the body's antioxidant defenses, but frequent hard exercise has the opposite effect, accelerating free-radical production well beyond the body's ability to cope. This can lead to dampened immunity, increased risk of heart disease and cancer, and premature aging.

a) very moderately—1

b) moderately—2

c) moderately hard—3

d) very hard—4

e) extremely hard—5

7. What is your general level of stress?

A stressful way of life also accelerates free-radical production.

a) mild—1

b) moderate—2

c) sometimes high, sometimes low—3

d) usually high—4

e) always high—5

8. How often each week do you eat deep-fried foods?

*While they may be delicious, deep-fried foods
are loaded with oxidized fats, which enhance
free-radical activity in your body.*

a) 1 or fewer times—1

b) 2 times—2

c) 3 times—3

d) 4 times—4

e) 5 times or more—5

9. How many times a week do you eat sugary
   junk food?

   *High-sugar foods increase your chances of
   developing type 2 diabetes, which accelerates free-radical production dramatically.
   They also raise levels of stress hormones and
   hamper immune system activity.*

   a) 1 or fewer times—1

   b) 2 times—2

   c) 3 times—3

   d) 4 times—4

   e) 5 times or more—5

10. How many times a week do you eat charred
    meat?

    *Meat cooked over a flame contains abundant
    free radicals and carcinogens.*

    a) 1 or fewer times—1

    b) 2 times—2

    c) 3 times—3

    d) 4 times—4

    e) 5 times or more—5

11. How many times per year do you catch a cold
    or the flu?

    *When you are sick with a cold or flu virus,
    your body creates more free radicals; a weak*

immune system is a good indication that you are not getting enough antioxidant nutrition.

a) 1 or fewer times—1

b) 2 times—2

c) 3 times—3

d) 4 times—4

e) 5 times or more—5

12. Do you have allergies or asthma?

Chronic inflammation—which these conditions signify—creates extra free-radical burden in the body.

a) no—1   b) yes—5

13. Do you have high LDL and low HDL cholesterol?

If so, you'll need to be sure you are getting enough antioxidants to slow the process of LDL oxidation.

a) no—1   b) yes—5

14. Do you have type 2 diabetes? (If you don't but it runs in your family, choose b.)

High blood sugar strongly accelerates oxidation throughout the body.

a) no—1   b) runs in family—3   c) yes—5

15. Do you have heart disease or a history of stroke? (If you don't but it runs in your family, choose b.)

Antioxidants protect against circulatory disease in many ways. For instance, vitamin E reduces LDL oxidation and inflammation and helps to keep blood vessels open, and vitamin C strengthens blood vessel walls.

a) no—1   b) runs in family—3   c) yes—5

16. Do you have cancer? (If you don't but it runs in your family, choose b; if you have had cancer in the past, choose c.)

    There is good evidence that excess free radicals are one of the root causes of cancer, and that high doses of antioxidants are an important part of healing from this disease.

    a) no—1

    b) runs in family—2

    c) I have had cancer but do not have it now—4

    d) I have cancer—5

17. Do you have rheumatoid arthritis or another autoimmune condition? (If members of your family do but you don't, choose b.)

    Like allergies and asthma, these conditions involve excess inflammation, which involves excess free-radical production.

    a) no—1   b) runs in family—3   c) yes—5

18. Do you have pale eyes (blue, gray, or green)?

    Age-related eye diseases such as cataracts and macular degeneration are caused by oxidative damage to the lens and retina. Light-colored eyes lend less protection against UV rays than dark eyes.

    a) no, I have dark eyes—1

    b) yes, and I am careful about protecting them from the sun—3

    c) yes, and I go without sunglasses—5

19. Do you live in a polluted area? Choose "e" for most polluted (urban) areas; choose "a" for least polluted; rank your area somewhere in between if you live in the suburbs.

Air (indoor and outdoor) and other types of pollutants enhance free-radical production in the body. Also take into account your day-to-day exposure to chemicals, such as pesticides, herbicides, household cleansers, solvents, and so on.

a) 1 (least polluted)

b) 2

c) 3

d) 4

e) 5 (most polluted)

Calculate Your Score

Add up the points you scored on each question.

If your total is between 20 and 40, excellent! You are not subjected to a great deal of oxidative stress, and you will probably not need more than a few basic antioxidant nutrients in dosages that can be found in a high-quality daily multivitamin and mineral supplement.

If you score between 41 and 60, you're still in good shape. You may need to ramp up the types and dosages of antioxidants you use from time to time, to deal with illness, high stress, or increased exposure to pollutants.

A score between 61 and 80 is not so good. You may want to consider a more intense program of antioxidant supplementation, with a wider range of nutrients and higher doses of each.

Finally, if you scored between 81 and 95, you are at high risk of excessive free-radical stress and the chronic disease states that are associated with this stress. Pay close attention to the nutrient pre-scriptions in the chapters to come. Antioxidants could very well turn your health around.

CHAPTER 3

ANTIOXIDANT VITAMINS AND MINERALS

In the 1890s, Dutch physician Christiaan Eijkman found his niche in Java studying the disease *beriberi*—a condition that could cause weight loss, emotional disturbances, impairments in sensory perception, weakness, and heartbeat irregularities. At that time, in Java, beriberi was not at all uncommon.

Dr. Eijkman found that chickens who were fed a steady diet of polished rice, from which the fiber-rich husks had been removed, displayed symptoms much like those seen in humans with beriberi. Feeding them the rice husks cured them rapidly. Dr. Eijkman then successfully used the same nutritional therapy to treat humans with beriberi and wrote about his findings.

A couple of decades later, around the year 1912, Polish biochemist Casimir Funk read Eijkman's work and attempted to isolate the substance in rice husks that cured beriberi. He was successful, and called his discovery *thiamine,* or *vitamin B$_1$—"vita"* meaning "life," and *"amine"* meaning that the substance contained an amine group. Funk rightly hypothesized that some other nutrient would probably turn out to be the cure for scurvy, a disease that commonly killed two-thirds or more of the men on long sea voyages. That antiscorbutic vitamin turned out to be vitamin C.

Since Casimir Funk's day, many more vitamins have been discovered. And since that time when they were used simply to cure deficiency diseases—which they did very rapidly, bringing people back from death's door to a decent state of health in a matter of hours—vitamin therapy has come a long, long way.

Antioxidant vitamins—particularly, vitamin C and vitamin E—have been the subjects of a great deal of study. The use of high supplemental doses of vitamins C and E is a safe and effective way to reduce the impact of aging on the body. Since 1951, nearly 22,500 peer-reviewed scientific studies involving vitamin E's effects on health have been published in medical journals; in the same amount of time, nearly 10,000 such studies involving vitamin C have been published. The scientific evidence to support the use of vitamin C and vitamin E for longer, healthier life—and for the prevention of Alzheimer's disease, cancer, and heart disease—is solid.

Vitamin C: The All-Purpose Antioxidant

In the late 1960s, two-time Nobel laureate Linus Pauling, Ph.D., began to publicly recommend the use of high doses of vitamin C (also known as ascorbate or ascorbic acid) to reduce cold and flu symptoms. Several years later, he reported on the research he and colleague Ewan Cameron had done on end-stage cancer patients. They found that giving patients 10 grams of vitamin C per day intravenously had remarkable effects on the survival time of these patients, some of whom lived for years even though they were expected to live only a few months. The high-dose of vitamin C also helped to reduce the severe pain that end-stage cancer patients typically experience.

More recently, a research team from Cambridge University recruited almost 19,500 subjects aged forty-five to seventy-nine for a vitamin C study. The participants filled out a questionnaire at the study's outset, describing their diet and lifestyle in detail. Vitamin C levels in the blood were periodically measured, and whenever a study subject died, the cause of death was recorded. After four years, it was found that the group with the highest vitamin C levels were half as likely to die from any cause as the group with the lowest levels. Men and women with low levels of vitamin C were more likely to end up with heart disease, while high vitamin C appeared to protect the men against cancer. The scientists concluded that a single extra serving of a vitamin C–rich vegetable or fruit, containing 30 to 250 milligrams of vitamin C, was associated with a 20 percent decrease in risk of death during the four-year-long study.

Some vitamin C experts believe that our inability to manufacture this nutrient in our bodies is the result of an evolutionary fluke. Of all the mammals that walk, swim, or fly, we are among a select few that do not make vitamin C from glucose in our livers, and so we must take it in on a regular basis. (Other primates are in the same boat, but they live on vitamin C–rich plants, so they get plenty.) Animals that make vitamin C make a great deal of it in proportion to their body weight: the equivalent of 10 to 12 grams for a human! In light of this fact, the adult RDA (recommended daily allowance) of 60 to 100 milligrams per day is, to say the least, scanty. Also inadequate is the average person's intake: for example, more than one-third of 500 patients at clinics in Phoenix, Arizona, were found to have low blood levels of this all-important antioxidant vitamin.

As mentioned above, vitamin C is also known as *ascorbic acid.* Ascorbic acid to which magnesium or calcium have been bound is called magnesium *ascorbate* or calcium *ascorbate.* This type of binding buffers vitamin C's acidity, which may be necessary to avoid digestive irritation when high doses of the nutrient are used. Vitamin C easily donates electrons to free radicals, including the *hydroxyl, superoxide,* and *hypochlorite* radicals. It is especially good at protecting LDL cholesterol against oxidation. It also works cooperatively with vitamin E, donating electrons to "spent" vitamin E molecules that have become free radicals themselves in the process of donating their own electrons. This free-radical-busting action of vitamin C is only one of the several functions it has in the body, not all of which are completely understood.

Many biochemical reactions require the participation of vitamin C, including the synthesis of *collagen*, the connective tissue from which bone, skin, blood vessels, and muscles are built; and the optimal activation of the immune system in the face of colds, flu viruses, and infections. Here are a few other ways in which vitamin C protects and promotes good health:

- Doses of 500 milligrams per day can reduce blood pressure by up to 10 percent, according to two recent studies.

- Vitamin C supplements have been found to help reverse *endothelial dysfunction*—stiffness and contractedness along the blood vessels caused by diets high in saturated fats and refined carbohydrates. Supplementation of 1 gram (1,000 milligrams) of vitamin C per day improves blood vessel flexibility. (The addition of vitamin E enhances this effect.)

- Several studies have found that vitamin C protects against stroke as well as brain damage from stroke.

- High doses (1,000 to 10,000 milligrams a day) help the body resist the flu. Two Salt Lake City chiropractors had forty-seven patients take 1,000 milligrams of vitamin C per hour for six hours as soon as they first felt flu symptoms coming on. Twenty-three patients got symptom relief within the first six hours; nineteen got relief with two six-hour treatments; and five got relief with three six-hour treatments.

- Linus Pauling was right—vitamin C does help cure the common cold! A professor at the University of Helsinki, Finland, found in his analysis of twenty-one studies that 2 to 6 grams of vitamin C per day reduced cold symptoms by about one-third.

- Creams rich in vitamin C have been found to reduce fine wrinkles and roughness in aging skin, as well as to generally improve skin tone and complexion.

- Vitamin C supplements may help prevent osteoporosis. A study of middle-aged and elderly women found that those who took vitamin C supplements had much greater bone density than those who did not.

Eat Foods Rich In Vitamin C and Take Your Supplements!

While you can't achieve daily vitamin C intake of 500 or more milligrams a day without supplements, it's still important to get as much of this nutrient as possible from foods. Red chili peppers, guava, sweet red and green peppers, kale, parsley, leafy greens, broccoli, watercress, cauliflower, persimmons, red cabbage, strawberries, papaya, and spinach are all rich in vitamin C. Oranges contain less, but they're still a good source, especially if you eat the whole orange with the white cuticle—a superior source of *bioflavonoids*, another nutrient that helps the body absorb and utilize vitamin C (more on flavonoids in Chapter 5). Keep in mind that the vitamin C in foods is destroyed by heating, and that vitamin C is quickly lost after harvesting or slicing. It follows that you should eat foods rich in this vitamin as soon as possible after they come from the fields or orchards, with a minimum of preparation.

You have plenty of choices when it comes to supplementation. You can take tablets, capsules, or chewables; you can mix powdered ascorbic acid or ascorbate in juice or water and drink it down. Chewables aren't a good idea if you plan to take 1,000 milligrams or more a day, because the acidity can wear down tooth enamel.

Most experts recommend at least 1,000 milligrams per day for generally healthy people, increasing the dosage whenever you are stressed or feel an illness coming on. Dosages higher than this might cause diarrhea; if you find this happens to you, back off of the dose until it goes away. It is believed that reaching your *bowel tolerance level*—the dosage at which you develop diarrhea—is a sign that you have gone just beyond your body's vitamin C requirement, and stepping back 1,000 milligrams a day from that dose will put you at your perfect dosage level.

If you feel any gastrointestinal distress from ascorbic acid, switch to a buffered (ascorbate) form. High doses—beyond 5,000 milligrams per day—are best taken as powder mixed with liquid. If you are a cancer patient or have some other serious health condition and would like to try high-dose intravenous vitamin C, consult with your doctor.

Vitamin E: Heart Protector

In the 1940s, Canadian physicians Wilfrid and Evan Shute discovered that supplements containing natural vitamin E could reverse heart disease. The rewards they reaped for this discovery were similar to those reaped by other pioneers in the field of nutritional research: they were scoffed at and doubted by a medical establishment that refused to believe that such a simple, natural therapy could be so effective against the number-one killer in North America.

The brothers Shute continued to recommend vitamin E supplements to their patients, and now, decades after their deaths, it has come to be recognized as a highly effective heart disease preventative. Cardiologists and general practitioners alike routinely recommend vitamin E supplementation to help their patients avoid heart attack.

Probably the most striking proof of the heart-protective effects of this antioxidant comes from a study by Nigel G. Stephens, M.D., and his coworkers at Cambridge University in England. He gave 400 or 800 IU (international units) of natural vitamin E or placebo to 2,000 patients with previously diagnosed heart disease. Compared to the placebo group, the vitamin E users reduced their incidence of heart attack by an amazing 77 percent!

Vitamin E: Protector of Polyunsaturated Fatty Acids (Pufas) and Anti-Inflammatory

In scientific parlance, vitamin E is regarded as the major chain-breaking antioxidant located in cell membranes. In plain English: vitamin E is a part of the fatty membranes that surround all cells, and it quenches several types of free radicals, stopping oxidative chain reactions. The more *polyunsaturated fatty acids* (PUFAs) are found in a cell membrane, the more vitamin E that cell requires to prevent free-radical damage. PUFAs make cell membranes flexible. They facilitate the passge of nutrients into the cell and wastes out of the cell. Vitamin E specializes in protecting these delicate fatty acids against oxidation. Cells with particularly high PUFA levels include *erythrocytes* (red blood cells), *neurons* (the cells of the nervous system), and the *epithelium* (lining) of the lungs.

Immune cells that engulf *pathogens* (disease-causing agents) also require plenty of vitamin E to protect them against the oxidation that occurs when they kill off an unwanted invader. Vitamin E may also play a crucial role in modulating the signaling pathways that allow cells to communicate with one another.

In order to fully understand the role of vitamin E as an antioxidant, we need to revisit the link between inflammation and oxidation. In Chapter 1, we explained how free-radical stress and inflammation interact to transform LDL cholesterol into hazardous material that causes swollen plaques to develop along the walls of blood vessels.

Recently, a new test has been developed to measure heart disease risk: a test that measures *C-reactive protein (CRP)* levels in the bloodstream. C-reactive protein is a marker of inflammation. Studies by Paul Ridker, M.D., of Harvard Medical School have revealed that high levels of CRP in the blood increase the likelihood of heart attack by four and a half times.

Other research has shown that high doses of vitamin E reliably lowers CRP levels. Researchers at the University of Otago, New Zealand, showed that CRP levels were lowered by half in subjects who took 800 IU of vitamin E for four weeks. (Vitamin C and lycopene did not have the same effects.) In another study, seventy-two subjects were asked to take 1,200 IU of vitamin E per day for three months. Some were diabetic, some had heart disease, and some were healthy. In all three groups, levels of CRP fell an average of 30 percent and levels of another inflammatory marker—the "parent" of CRP, called *interleukin-6*—fell 50 percent.

Vitamin E has other anti-inflammatory effects, including inhibition of *COX-2*, a substance made in the body that exacerbates inflammation; inhibition of adhesion molecules, which promote inflammation; and the "turning off" of genes that can cause the normal, healing inflammatory response to spiral out of control.

The anti-inflammatory effects of vitamin E help to explain why it has healing effects on people with *rheumatoid arthritis (RA)*, a painful runaway inflammation of joint tissues. A study published in the *Annals of the Rheumatic Diseases* demonstrated that 900 IU of vitamin E per day twice daily reduced RA pain by about 50 percent, and 60 percent of the patients taking vitamin E reported feeling better overall during the course of the twelve-week study.

Respiratory allergies may also respond well to vitamin E. A study from the University of Nottingham in England revealed that those whose diets were richer in vitamin E had lower levels of *immunoglobulin E, or IgE.* IgE is a marker of allergic reactions. Animal studies have replicated this result and illustrated that high dietary vitamin E intake reduces blood concentrations of pro-inflammatory proteins called *cytokines.*

Vitamin E Protects Against Exercise-Induced Free-Radical Damage

In the 1970s, studies performed at the University of California, Davis, showed that exercise increased lipid peroxidation, especially in a high-ozone environment like that of cities all over the world. High doses of vitamin E proved effective in reducing this lipid peroxidation.

Lipid Peroxidation
The damaging effects of free radicals on fats.

More recently, German researchers analyzed blood samples from men who had just run until exhausted on a treadmill. They found considerable DNA damage compared to samples taken before the run. Multivitamin supplements actually increased DNA damage, most likely because of the free-radical-catalyzing effects of the copper and iron in the supplements. It was found that 1,600 IU of vitamin E, given in two doses on the day before the test, plus 800 IU the day after, reduced DNA damage. Finally, the researchers gave subjects 1,200 IU of vitamin E per day for two weeks before the treadmill workout, and this prevented all DNA damage in four of the five subjects and reduced it in the fifth. Their study was published in the April 1995 issue of the journal *Mutation Research*.

Vitamin E, Selenium, and Prostate Cancer

At this writing, a large clinical trial designed to determine the effects of vitamin E (400 IU/day) and selenium (200 micrograms/day) on men's risk of developing prostate cancer is underway.

Prostate cancer affects one in six men and is the second most common cancer in American males. So far, the results of this trial—dubbed SELECT (Selenium and Vitamin E Chemoprevention Trial)—indicate that this combination of nutrients does indeed protect the prostate gland against cancerous transformation.

Selenium
An essential mineral that participates in several of the body's antioxidant defense systems. It and vitamin E form a component of glutathione peroxidase.

Helping to set the foundation for SELECT were two earlier studies. In a 1996 study, men and women took selenium to prevent nonmelanoma skin cancer; they did not decrease their risk of skin cancer, but the men had 60 percent fewer cases of prostate cancer. In another study in 1998, Finnish researchers gave either vitamin E or a placebo to 29,100 male smokers. The vitamin E users had 32 percent fewer cases of prostate cancer during the course of the study.

Vitamin E, Alzheimer's Disease, and Diabetes

Alzheimer's disease (AD) causes characteristic changes in the brain. Deposits of a substance called *beta-amyloid* have been linked with Alzheimer's, although it is not clear whether it is a cause or an effect of the disease. Beta-amyloid, in turn, has been linked to excessive oxidation in the brain, and free-radical activity is now believed to be a major contributor to AD. Research has demonstrated consistently that high vitamin E intake through foods can lower the risk of AD, but the use of this nutrient hasn't been widely recommended for the prevention of this disease. Some studies of vitamin E supplementation have failed to show significant benefit in AD prevention.

The same has been true of diabetes: it is accepted as scientific fact that free-radical overload plays a major role in adult-onset (type 2) diabetes, and higher intake of vitamin E has been linked with lowered risk of developing this disease. Diets rich in antioxidant nutrients have been found to help protect against diabetes and diabetes complications. But antioxidant supplementation studies haven't been very compelling. Why? *Because most of the studies on antioxidant supplementation have used only one nutrient at a time.* Antioxidants don't occur this way in nature. They need one another to do their work in the body.

Antioxidant Nutrients Work Cooperatively

Those who try to design studies to prove the benefits of specific antioxidant nutrients face a catch-22: High doses of single nutrients often don't have the benefits we think they should have, because these nutrients are designed to work cooperatively with other nutrients. But when scientists try to do studies that incorporate more than one nutrient, they are accused of being unscientific—of not isolating the effects of each nutrient so that their actions can be better understood.

Vitamin E is "recycled" by vitamin C and *glutathione*, an antioxidant that is endogenous, or made in the body (see Chapter 4 for more on glutathione). When vitamin E scavenges a free radical, it is then itself oxidized—that is, missing an electron. Vitamin C and glutathione donate electrons to vitamin E, renewing its antioxidant power.

This kind of synergy happens on a larger scale between many of the other antioxidant substances that will be addressed in this book.

Remember those studies that put a scare into antioxidant users by suggesting that certain antioxidants might, in fact, *cause* diseases related to free-radical stress—namely, cancer? One study with such findings was on beta-carotene in smokers; another, a test-tube study of vitamin C, suggested that high doses might cause damage to DNA. The outcomes of these studies were directly related to an imbalanced intake of antioxidant nutrients, which can create heightened oxidation in the body in the long run.

Let's look at a few studies that illustrate the synergy of the antioxidant vitamins C and E.

Vitamins C and E Protect Against Reperfusion Injury

Much of the damage that occurs in a person who survives a heart attack or *occlusive stroke*—where a blood vessel in the brain is clogged and constricted by cholesterol-filled plaques—is the result of *reperfusion injury.* Blood flow is temporarily stopped to a part of the heart or brain, and when that blood flow is restored, there is a rush of free-radical production that can't be dealt with through the body's natural antioxidant defenses. According to one recent study by researchers at Columbia University, the oxidized form of vitamin C— *dehydroascorbic acid,* which can be converted back to vitamin C when it is reduced by another antioxidant, such as vitamin E—was found to pass easily through the blood-brain barrier in lab mice. When given before a stroke, the dehydroascorbic acid prevented up to 95 percent of damage! These results were so striking that the researchers recommended that vitamin C be used as a drug to treat stroke patients.

Vitamins E and C Effective Against Alzheimer's Disease

A study published in the January 2004 issue of *Archives of Neurology* reported the results of vitamin E and C supplementation in a group of 3,200 residents of Cache County, Utah, who were over sixty-five years of age. The researchers found that 185 of the participants had dementia and 104 had early-stage Alzheimer's disease. Participants were asked about their supplement use, and it turned out that those who used a combination of vitamins C and E were least likely to have Alzheimer's disease. Subjects who took vitamin E or C alone, B complex alone, or a combination of vitamin C and multivitamins did not reduce their risk of Alzheimer's, but those who took vitamin E plus multivitamins or E and C without multivitamins had the lowest risk of the disease.

Choosing the Right Vitamin E Supplement

Although vitamin E is generally regarded as a single nutrient, it actually is a designation given to a family of eight related compounds. These compounds are divided into two categories, the *tocopherols* and the *tocotrienols*. Alpha-tocopherol has the greatest antioxidant activity, followed by beta tocopherol. Next in line for antioxidant potency is alpha-tocotrienol; then, gamma-tocopherol; and last but not least, delta-tocopherol. Alpha- and gamma-tocopherols are most commonly found in foods.

It has generally been recognized that alpha-tocopherol (in its natural form, d-alpha-tocopherol, and not the synthetic dl-alpha-tocopherol) is the best one to take in supplement form. More recent data suggest, however, that only using alpha-tocopherol could deplete the body of gamma-tocopherol, which these recent studies show may be an even better cancer preventative and anti-inflammatory than alpha-tocopherol.

At this point, the best way to go is to use a natural vitamin E supplement that contains alpha- and gamma-tocopherols, and some of the other tocopherols and tocotrienols, as well. Healthy people can try 400 to 800 IU a day. If you have heart disease, cancer, or a chronic inflammatory condition, you may want to try taking more; do so with the guidance of a nutritionally oriented physician. Vitamin E is a potent blood thinner, so be sure to stop using it a couple of weeks before having surgery, and don't take high doses if you use anticlotting medication.

Take vitamin E with food that contains fat for best absorption. If you take fish oil supplements, take them along with your vitamin E.

Special Forms of Vitamin E for Breast Cancer

Studies of a natural form of vitamin E called *alpha-tocopherol succinate* has been found to inhibit the growth of breast cancer cells in test-tube studies. The tocotrienols, however, seem to have the most significant potential both to slow the growth of breast cancer tumors and to reduce the chances that cancerous cells will form in the breasts in the first place.

Test-tube studies of estrogen-receptor-positive breast cancer cells have found that tocotrienols can inhibit the growth of these cells by as much as 50 percent. This inhibitory effect is seen at low concentrations of tocotrienols, compared to the amount of alpha-tocopherol succinate required to inhibit breast cancer growth. Test-tube studies have demonstrated that tocotrienols cause breast cancer cell *apoptosis* (cell death).

Other studies indicate that palm oil tocopherols, when added to the breast cancer drug tamoxifen in a breast-cancer-cell culture, dramatically improves the effectiveness of the drug. In one study, tamoxifen alone reduced estrogen-receptor-positive breast cancer cell growth by 50 percent, but when tocotrienols were added, a 95 percent growth inhibition was seen. Tocotrienols also have been found to reduce the dose of tamoxifen needed to inhibit breast cancer growth—a good thing, considering the side effects this drug can have. (Similar studies found that alpha-tocopherol actually increases the tamoxifen requirement for slowing of breast-cancer-cell growth, which might indicate that women with breast cancer who are on tamoxifen may want to avoid taking high doses of alpha-tocopherol alone.)

How much tocotrienol should you take to prevent or slow breast cancer growth? According to a review of current research by the Life Extension Foundation, around 90 milligrams (roughly equivalent to 90 IU) is probably enough to raise blood and breast tocotrienol concentrations significantly. You can take up to 240 milligrams a day safely.

CHAPTER 4

ANTIOXIDANTS
MADE IN THE BODY

Most informed vitamin users know about the antioxidant vitamins; some know that minerals can also be indispensable when it comes to fighting free-radical damage. Many people have heard of antioxidant *phytochemicals*—non-vitamin, non-mineral plant chemicals—found in foods and herbs, and we'll fill you in on the best of those later in this book. But what people *don't* generally know is that their bodies make their own antioxidant substances to deal with the constant metabolic production of free radicals.

Until recently, there wasn't much focus in the nutrition news about these *endogenous antioxidants*—antioxidants that are made in the body. The most likely reason for this is the following logic: If we can't increase the activity of those antioxidants, as we can increase levels of antioxidant vitamins and minerals in our bodies through good diet and supplementation, why give them any press? Better we should focus on what we can control, right?

Yes and no. It turns out that the body's production of endogenous antioxidants—including coenzyme Q_{10}, glutathione, and alpha-lipoic acid—*can* be supplemented, and that this can produce dramatic benefit. Even though our bodies make these substances, adding more to the mix with prudent supplementation can make a big difference in our health.

Our cells make less of these endogenous antioxidants as we get older. This decrease in endogenous antioxidant protection is considered to be a significant contributor to aging and to the onset of chronic age-related diseases. There is good evidence that boosting cellular levels of natural antioxidants with supplements could help control or prevent age-related diseases—including heart disease, cancer, diabetes, and Alzheimer's disease.

Coenzyme Q_{10}: Key Element of Metabolism

Within each of the cells of your body, tiny "engines" called *mitochondria* work night and day to produce energy from the carbohydrates and fats you take in through your diet. It's hard to imagine that bagel you ate this morning ending up as carbohydrate molecules that are being transformed into *adenosine triphosphate* (*ATP*), the energy currency of the body; however, this process—known as *metabolism*—is what powers your body at the cellular level. Think of ATP as little energy packets that are broken apart (into adenosine diphosphate and a single phosphate) wherever energy is required.

Metabolism is a mind-boggling, complex process, as you well know if you ever sat through a mammalian physiology class in college. Dozens of biochemical reactions are involved, and *enzymes* participate in each of those reactions. Without enzymes, metabolism would very quickly cease.

Enzymes
Proteins that accelerate the rate at which chemical reactions occur.

Similarly important are the *coenzymes*, which work alongside the enzymes to enable them to perform their various functions. Most of the B vitamins, many of the minerals, and vitaminlike *quinones* (biologically important compounds) are coenzymes. One such quinone is *ubiquinone*—one of the scientific names for coenzyme Q_{10} (CoQ_{10} for short).

Related compounds are found in plant cells (plastoquinones) and even in bacteria (menaquinones). CoQ_{10} is found in each and every animal cell, which explains why its scientific name, ubiquinone, has the same root as the word "ubiquitous." The higher the energy requirements of an organ, the higher the concentration of CoQ_{10}.

Within the walls of the heart, which work constantly from your twelfth week in your mother's uterus and throughout the rest of your days, Co Q_{10} concentrations are twice that of other muscles in the body. The kidneys and liver work overtime to neutralize and get rid of toxins; these organs also contain high concentrations of CoQ_{10}. Research shows us that people with heart disease or with kidney or liver disease have low CoQ_{10} levels; a deficiency of this nutrient would naturally strike first and hardest in these organs.

CoQ_{10} Levels Decrease with Age and Illness

CoQ_{10} production peaks at about the age of twenty. By our eighties, most of our CoQ_{10} levels will have fallen by 65 percent. To make CoQ_{10}, our cells require several B vitamins and trace minerals, as well as vitamin C; if we don't take in adequate amounts of these nutrients, we're at even greater risk of not having enough of this endogenous antioxidant to go around. Statin drugs (HMG-CoA reductase inhibitors) such as Pravachol and lovastatin are widely prescribed for cholesterol control, but they deplete CoQ_{10} production significantly, which is bad for heart health in the long run. Poor diet, chronic stress, and extremely hard exercise also drain CoQ_{10} reserves.

Some experts claim that CoQ_{10}'s antioxidant power far exceeds that of vitamin E. It works alongside vitamin E, renewing alpha-tocopherol when it has become a free radical itself. Like vitamin E, it protects lipids (fats) and proteins against peroxidation by free radicals, including the LDL cholesterol that floats around in the bloodstream.

CoQ_{10} is most highly concentrated along the inner membrane of the mitochondria, where free radicals are produced during metabolism. CoQ_{10} also protects the cells against the burst of free radicals that is produced when white blood cells respond to invasion by bacteria.

CoQ_{10} *Is a Heart-Smart Antioxidant*

The more advanced a person's heart disease, the lower their level of CoQ_{10}. This association has inspired researchers to look closely at the ways in which CoQ_{10} protects and promotes heart health.

When CoQ_{10} becomes depleted in the heart muscle, the results may take years to manifest. Slight lack of this nutrient is believed to cause, over time, microscopic damage to the heart muscle and the coronary arteries (the vessels that feed the heart muscle), as unquenched free radicals are released throughout and out of the mitochondria.

During a heart attack, there is an explosion of free radicals that can cause extensive damage to the heart muscle. When blood flow is abruptly restored through an artery that has become clogged, reperfusion injury can result, causing damage to the heart muscle that weakens its pumping capacity.

In one study, researchers pretreated rats with CoQ_{10}, then isolated their living, beating hearts and experimentally created a heart attack in each one. After twenty-five minutes of *ischemia* (lack of blood flow to a part of the heart muscle due to a constricted vessel), the hearts were allowed to reperfuse (fill with oxygenated blood) for forty more minutes. Compared to another group of rats that were given salt solution instead of CoQ_{10}, the CoQ_{10} rats had less oxidative damage to their heart mitochondria. The researchers concluded that a period of CoQ_{10} supplementation could significantly aid the heart muscle's ability to bounce back from a heart attack.

Another study, this one by German researchers, evaluated the effects of selenium and CoQ_{10} treatment in sixty-one human heart attack patients. Thirty-two of them received 500 micrograms (mcg) of selenium soon after their heart attack, and 100 milligrams (mg) of CoQ_{10} and 100 mcg of selenium daily for a year following. The other half of the patients received placebo preparations. After a year, an electrocardiogram showed no lengthening of the QT interval—an indication of heart damage—in the group using selenium and Co Q_{10}, while in the other group, 40 percent had QT lengthening. During the follow-up, 20 percent of the control group (a total of six people) died from a heart attack, while only one person in the antioxidant group died—of noncardiac causes.

CoQ_{10} has the capacity to prevent heart attacks, too. In animal models of *atherosclerosis* (the process whereby inflamed plaques build up in the coronary arteries), CoQ_{10} was found to inhibit the formation of atherosclerotic lesions.

CoQ_{10} for Heart Failure

The most intensively studied use for CoQ_{10} is as an aid to heart failure patients. A heart that has been weakened to the point of not having enough "oomph" to pump adequate blood through the cardiovascular system, heart failure is a common consequence of heart attack or viral heart disease. In the early 1980s, Karl Folkers, Ph.D., and Per H. Langsjoen, M.D., conducted the first study using CoQ_{10} to treat heart failure. Their subjects, nineteen patients who had previously been expected to die from heart failure, rebounded with "extraordinary clinical improvement" when given CoQ_{10}.

In a later study by Dr. Langsjoen, 806 heart failure and ischemic heart disease patients were treated by 65 cardiologists. The overall impression was that CoQ_{10} offered significant benefits. Another study compared 319 patients on CoQ_{10} with 322 who took placebo; the CoQ_{10} reduced complications of heart failure and the need for hospitalization. Finally, a study of 2,500 heart failure patients at 173 medical centers in Italy were given 50–150 mg of CoQ_{10} per day for three months, and 80 percent showed some type of improvement.

Overall, the research shows that CoQ_{10} supplementation in heart attack patients reduces angina (heart pains), irregular heart rhythms, and free-radical stress in the heart muscle, and that it improves the heart's pumping strength. The number of cardiac deaths and nonfatal heart attacks is reduced in heart attack survivors who take CoQ_{10}. CoQ_{10} has also been found to help reduce high blood pressure, a major risk factor for coronary artery disease.

CoQ_{10} and Statins: An Important Relationship

Statin drugs interfere with the production of cholesterol, but they also interfere with the production of CoQ_{10}. As the importance of this antioxidant to heart health is increasingly recognized, it's likely to become standard practice to supplement statin users—who number over 30 million at this writing, with more getting prescriptions every day—with a generous amount of Co Q_{10}. Evidence suggests that doing so will improve the benefit of the drugs, and will probably help to alleviate the fatigue that many statin users experience as a side effect.

CoQ_{10} for Cancer

Research into CoQ_{10}'s protective effects against cancer is still in its early stages. Preliminary evidence is promising, however.

CoQ_{10}, like most other antioxidants, appears

to protect DNA against oxidative damage. This action is believed to prevent the initial development of cancerous growths. There is also strong evidence that this nutrient can play a significant role in shrinking tumors that have already been established.

Danish cancer surgeon Knud Lockwood, M.D., gave thirty-two "high-risk" breast cancer patients a combination of CoQ_{10}, antioxidant vitamins, and essential fatty acids. According to his report in the March 30, 1994 issue of *Biochemical and Biophysical Research Communications,* "No patient died and all expressed a feeling of well-being . . . These clinical results are remarkable since about four deaths would have been expected. Now, after 24 months, all still survive; about six deaths would have been expected." Six of the subjects had partial remission of their tumors. One woman had a recurrence of her cancer following lumpectomy, and with doses of 390 mg per day of CoQ_{10}, the tumor disappeared!

Another patient, who was age seventy-four at the time, refused a second surgery when her cancer returned. After three months of 300 mg per day of CoQ_{10}, a mammogram and exam revealed no tumor or metastases (offshoots of the original tumor in other parts of the body). Dr. Lockwood writes in his article that, having treated some 7,000 cases of breast cancer over thirty-five years, he had never before seen "a spontaneous complete regression of a 1.5–2.0 centimeter breast tumor, and had never seen a comparable regression on any conventional anti-tumor therapy."

Levels of CoQ_{10} have been found to be low in women with cervical cancer. And a study of 200 women with breast cancer found a CoQ_{10} deficiency in cancerous and noncancerous lesions. The lower the concentration of CoQ_{10}, the worse the women's prognosis turned out to be.

CoQ_{10} appears to have immunity-enhancing

effects that may lend support to the body's natural defenses against cancer.

Other Benefits of CoQ$_{10}$

Diseased gum tissues—those that are afflicted with gingivitis or periodontitis—are low in CoQ$_{10}$. Anecdotal reports have revealed healing effects of CoQ$_{10}$ on diseased gums when it is swallowed or made into a mouth rinse.

Age spots are the result of mitochondrial dysfunction in skin cells. Topical CoQ$_{10}$ has become a cutting-edge method for staving off skin aging, and can be found in many skin-care products.

Neurodegenerative diseases—including Alzheimer's and Parkinson's diseases—have been linked with mitochondrial dysfunction and a resulting flaw in the ability of the nervous system's cells to produce adequate energy. Alzheimer's disease, in particular, has been associated with free-radical overload in the tissues of the brain. While none of the research indicates that CoQ$_{10}$ can prevent neurodegenerative diseases, there is evidence that supplementing this nutrient can slow the rate of cognitive decline in people with these diseases.

Chronic obstructive pulmonary disease (COPD) is characterized by chronic cough, difficult breathing, and wheezing. Like many chronically ill people, those with COPD have been found to have low CoQ$_{10}$ concentrations compared with healthy people. One study showed that patients with COPD had improved exercise tolerance when they took low doses of CoQ$_{10}$ (90 mg/day for eight weeks).

How Much CoQ$_{10}$ Should You Take?

It's virtually impossible to get meaningful amounts of CoQ$_{10}$ from foods. If you want to reap the benefits described in these pages, you will need to use a supplement. Whatever CoQ$_{10}$ you get from beef, fish, spinach, or nuts will help keep your cellular engines running smoothly, too.

For overall wellness, you can use between 10 and 150 mg a day. Doses ten times higher have been found to be safe, but there have been some reports of appetite loss, stomach inflammation, diarrhea, and nausea. Those with heart disease or cancer may want to consult with a physician about the best dose for them. The most effective daily dose in one Parkinson's disease study was 1,200 mg, and some heart patients may need 200–400 mg or more per day.

Because it is extremely fat soluble, CoQ_{10} is best absorbed in an oil-based form. The best forms are pre-dissolved in oil within a gelatin capsule. Dry, powdery CoQ_{10} can be sprinkled from the capsule over butter or nut butter for better absorption.

Alpha-Lipoic Acid: Versatile Antioxidant

In the February 2002 issue of the *Proceedings of the National Academy of Sciences*, the results of three studies were published—results that changed the minds of a lot of skeptics regarding the antiaging effects of targeted nutrient supplementation.

The studies were by a group of researchers from the University of California at Berkeley and the Children's Hospital of Oakland Research Institute. Bruce Ames—one of the original antioxidant researchers, the man for whom the Ames test for antioxidant activity is named—and coworkers gave rats a combination of two nutrients, *alpha-lipoic acid* and *acetyl-L-carnitine*. This combination had almost miraculous effects on aged rats, restoring them to a youthful state that amazed the research teams. Dr. Ames quipped that "with the two supplements together, these old rats got up and did the Macarena."

The rats were twenty to twenty-four months old

at the beginning of the study, which correlates to about seventy-five to eighty years of age in humans. When given the two supplements, the rats' performance on tests of memory improved; they became more active and energetic; their bodies' production of antioxidant substances rose; and their mitochondrial function improved.

In one of the three studies by Ames and colleagues, it was demonstrated that alpha-lipoic acid and acetyl-L-carnitine reduced oxidative damage and structural decay in the *hippocampus,* the part of the brain that deteriorates in Alzheimer's disease patients. Age-related memory loss is believed to be at least partly due to free-radical damage to the brain.

Acetyl-L-carnitine is a valuable supplement, but it does not have antioxidant activity that we know of. Here, we'll focus on the reasons why alpha-lipoic acid would have age-reversing effects on rats—and, by association, on people.

Alpha-Lipoic Acid (ALA) Overview

Mitochondria are the source of most of the free radicals produced in the body. They undergo a lot of wear and tear, and many scientists who study the aging process now believe that the oxidative decay of these organelles is the first step in the age-related breakdown of cellular function. In his research, Bruce Ames found that feeding acetyl-carnitine and lipoic acid—substances that are naturally occurring in the cells—we can slow the process of mitochondrial aging.

Like CoQ_{10}, ALA works as a coenzyme in the metabolic process within the mitochondria. Synthesized in the cells of both humans and plants, ALA contains two sulfur molecules, which can be either oxidized or reduced. ALA is a very powerful antioxidant in its own right, and can "recharge" vitamins C and E, as well as CoQ_{10} and glutathione, once they have reduced free radicals themselves. (ALA is the only antioxidant that's been proven to raise glutathione levels within the cells.) It is routinely converted to *dihydrolipoic acid,* a substance that possesses even greater antioxidant properties.

ALA's role in breaking down sugars (simple carbohydrates) for energy production has been known since 1951, but it was not until more than thirty years later that the antioxidant effects of ALA and dihydrolipoic acid were discovered.

Molecular and cellular biologist Lester Packer, Ph.D., a professor at the University of California at Berkeley, developed a checklist to evaluate the therapeutic value of antioxidants. According to Dr. Packer's checklist, the more of the following characteristics an antioxidant has, the more valuable it is for delaying age-related diseases:

- It is absorbed well in the gastrointestinal tract.

- It is converted within cells and tissues into more active antioxidant substances.

- It has antioxidant actions in lipids (for example, within the cell membrane) and aqueous (watery) regions of cells.

- It has low toxicity, so that doses needed to deliver improved antioxidant activity within the cells will not cause damage to those cells.

Not many antioxidants live up to all four of these criteria. Alpha-lipoic acid is one of the few that does. The catch is that only extra ALA—the amount above and beyond what is needed to maintain metabolic activity—will exert antioxidant effects. Supplementing the diet with ALA is really the only way to get enough into your body to stave off disease and increase life span. Some ALA is found in foods, but not enough to make any sizeable difference in your body's concentrations of this nutrient.

ALA is also a *chelator* of heavy metals, meaning that it helps to move excessive amounts of metals such as mercury, iron, aluminum, and copper safely out of the body. These metals are known to enhance the production of free radicals. Accumulation of aluminum and mercury in the tissues of the nervous system may turn out to be an important cause of Alzheimer's disease.

In test-tube studies, this nutrient prevented the activation of *nuclear factor kappa-B (NFK-B)*, a protein that can alter the behavior of genes. NFK-B has been implicated in the development of cancer and the replication of the HIV virus.

A process known as *glycation* has recently gained attention as a significant cause of cellular aging. Age spots on the skin are a visible sign of this process, which involves the binding together of sugars and proteins. Glycation is of particular concern in diabetics because of the chronically high levels of sugars that circulate in their bodies. Free radicals are produced fifty times faster by glycated proteins than by non-glycated proteins.

Alpha-lipoic acid has been found to prevent the formation of glycated proteins in test-tube studies. This could explain why ALA is proving to be such a valuable supplement for individuals with diabetes. In fact, ALA is widely used in Germany for the treatment of complications related to this disease.

ALA and Diabetes Complications

It has been known since 1970 that alpha-lipoic acid enhances the clearance of excess glucose from the bloodstream. More recent research shows that ALA helps to reverse insulin resistance and enhances the

Type 1 (Insulin-Dependent) Diabetes
When the body is unable to move glucose into the cells to be metabolized for energy because the pancreas does not make adequate insulin.

ability of insulin to move glucose into the cells—a crucial discovery for the treatment of both type 1 and type 2 diabetes. This disease dramatically increases the risk of coronary artery, kidney, and eye disease.

Type 2 (Non-Insulin-Dependent) Diabetes
When the cells develop a resistance to insulin, which then cannot move glucose to where it can be used as fuel.

Diabetic neuropathy, a common side effect of diabetes, is attributed to free-radical damage to nerves. It causes burning, sharp, cutting pain, prickly sensations, and—eventually, as the nerve tissue dies off—numbness. This is one reason why diabetics often end up with toes, feet, or legs amputated: they cannot feel small sores or abrasions on their toes, and by the time they are noticed, gangrene has set in.

Here is a sampling of the research into ALA and diabetic complications:

- *Diabetes Medicine* published a study that found that symptoms of pain, burning, and numbness decreased significantly after eight days of 600 mg of alpha-lipoic acid therapy administered by IV.

- The *Indian Journal of Medical Research* reported that alpha lipoic acid helped to reestablish a healthy oxidant/antioxidant balance in the liver and kidney of rats fed a high-fructose diet. These rats had quickly developed high insulin levels, increased lipid peroxides, and diminished endogenous antioxidant activity. ALA supplementation mitigated all of these ill effects of the diabetes-causing diet.

- Scientists in Russia and at the Mayo Clinic in the United States found that alpha-lipoic acid supplementation "significantly and rapidly reduces the frequency and severity of symptoms of the most common kind of diabetic neuropathy." The researchers found that lipoic acid actually improved the ability of nerves to conduct impulses.

- A study of twenty type 2 diabetics found that oral doses of 600, 1,200, and 1,800 mg of ALA daily for four weeks improved insulin sensitivity by 25 percent.

- A Canadian research group gave daily ALA to a portion of a group of rats genetically predisposed to diabetes and hypertension, and gave all of the study animals a diet containing 10 percent pure glucose. The rats who got glucose but no ALA had a 29 percent increase in blood pressure; a 30 percent increase in blood glucose; a 22 percent increase in the production of one type of free radical; a 286 percent increase in insulin levels; and a 408 percent increase in measurements of insulin resistance. The glycated protein levels of these unfortunate rats increased by 63 percent. The rats who got both ALA and glucose, however, had much smaller increases in their insulin levels and insulin resistance, and had no increases in glycation or production of the free radical that rose 22 percent in the non-ALA rats.

- Diabetics and those with insulin resistance are at greatly increased risk of coronary artery disease and occlusive stroke. A study from the Linus Pauling Institute shows that a combination of ALA and vitamin C increased the synthesis of *nitric oxide*, a natural blood vessel dilator, in the human aorta (a major blood vessel). This relaxing and expanding effect on blood vessels helps to prevent heart attack and stroke.

ALA and Brain Health

At the Central Institute for Mental Health in Germany, aged rats given ALA didn't do the Macarena. They did, however, perform better on tests of memory. Young mice given the same supplement did not show the same kind of improvements, which suggests that the older mice did better on the tests because something they had lost with the passage of time was being replaced.

ALA can also protect the brain against reperfusion injury following stroke. Researcher Manas Panigrahi, Ph.D., of the National Institute of Mental Health and Neurosciences in India, found that pretreatment with alpha-lipoic acid reduced the death rate from induced stroke to a third of that of animals that had not been pretreated. Research on reperfusion injury to the heart after a heart attack showed similar results.

Another German research group published their study of the anti-glycation effects of ALA, and how this might improve our odds of avoiding Alzheimer's disease. In their article for the December 2003 issue of the journal *Biochemical Society Transactions* titled "Anti-Aging Defenses against Alzheimer's Disease," these researchers write that "accumulation of insoluble protein deposits and their cross-linking by advanced glycation end products in the brain is a feature of aging and neurodegeneration, especially in Alzheimer's disease." By boosting the activity of glutathione (discussed in the next section) and through its own effects on the body, ALA may help to slow the oxidation that results from glycation; it can reduce glycation as well.

Researchers have also found that antioxidants such as ALA protect against mercury toxicity—a major issue these days due to the prevalence of methylmercury contamination in fish and the widespread use of mercury-containing dental amalgams. In a study by Swiss researchers, early onset Alzheimer's patients were found to have blood mercury levels three times higher than those of control subjects, while late-onset patients had levels twice that of controls.

Doses of 100–600 mg per day have been proven safe.

Glutathione: Antioxidant Detoxifier

Glutathione is, like the quinones, ubiquitous in living systems. It is so crucial to cellular health that its depletion within a cell leads to the death of that cell. Made up of three amino acids—L-glutamine, L-cysteine, and glycine—glutathione is a small molecule that exists in high concentrations throughout the body. It is most highly concentrated in the liver (at 10 millimoles) and is least concentrated in the blood plasma (4.5 micromoles). And glutathione happens to be one of the most powerful antioxidant agents known.

Glutathione protects cells by quenching some particularly dangerous forms of free radicals (including the hydroxyl radical). Its antioxidant power extends to protection of DNA against oxidative modification. It is the primary protectant of the eyes and skin against damaging ultraviolet (UV) radiation, and it is the foundation of the p450 detoxification system that neutralizes toxins in the liver, kidneys, lungs, and intestinal lining.

p450 Detoxification System

A series of enzymatic reactions that alters carcinogenic, or otherwise dangerous, substances, facilitating their removal from the body through urine or feces.

Glutathione also plays roles in the synthesis and repair of DNA, protein synthesis, amino acid transport, and the synthesis of hormonelike prostaglandins. It is also believed to play a role in immune system enhancement. Smoking, alcohol, caffeine, acetaminophen (sold as Tylenol), and some other drugs, vigorous exercise, ultraviolet radiation, air pollutants, and hormone-mimicking chemicals (xenobiotics) all deplete glutathione.

In people who are severely ill, glutathione levels are low. Aging leads to a reduction in glutathione production as well. Glutathione also supplies extra electrons to oxidized vitamin C. It is a component of the *glutathione peroxidases,* a group of selenium-containing enzymes that have wide-ranging antioxidant effects, and of the *glutathione S-transferases,* a family of multi-functional enzymes that join to toxins, including xenobiotics (chemical compounds, such as drugs). This makes the toxins easier to move out of the cell and out of the body. Glutathione seems like a natural choice for the prevention of age-related diseases, and it has been studied as a therapy for cancer, heart disease, and for the slowing of the natural aging process, and for support of immunity against viral illness.

Glutathione Research

The following are some highlights of the research on glutathione:

- In one animal study, liver cancers induced by the toxic mold *aflatoxin* regressed and survival was enhanced with glutathione administration. The survival difference was remarkable: all rats without supplemental glutathione died within twenty-four months, but 81 percent of the rats given glutathione survived past twenty-four months.

- A study of women with ovarian cancer showed a reduced rate of side effects and prolonged survival time with glutathione administered intravenously.

- Research published in the *New England Journal of Medicine* suggests that low glutathione levels may increase risk of heart attack.

- Glutathione concentrations are correlated with the body's ability to fight viruses, including AIDS.

- Inhalation of glutathione shows some promise as a treatment of respiratory diseases.

Why You Should Not
Take Glutathione Supplements

The catch is that glutathione is not absorbed well when taken orally. Some research suggests that it is soaked up by the cells along the intestinal wall and remains there.

The most reliable way to get glutathione into the circulation and into the cells is to take its precursors—the amino acids from which it is made. Cysteine, in a form called *N-acetylcysteine,* appears to be the best choice for this purpose. Alpha-lipoic acid, too, enhances glutathione production, but not as dramatically.

N-Acetylcysteine (NAC):
Glutathione Booster

Virtually every hospital emergency room in the United States stocks this nutrient, N-acetylcysteine (NAC), as an antidote for acetaminophen poisoning. When a person takes too much of the drug acetaminophen, the liver's supply of glutathione is quickly depleted. If glutathione runs out before the drug is detoxified, liver damage or liver failure is the end result. If large doses of NAC are given in time, liver glutathione is restored and the overdose can be broken down.

Since the 1960s, NAC has been used as a *mucolytic* agent. It helps to thin mucous secretions in those with cystic fibrosis and chronic bronchitis. Its rich store of sulfhydryl groups—which also happen to quench free radicals—gives NAC a unique ability to break the disulfide bonds of thick mucus, making it easier to move out of the body.

NAC is the principal rate-limiting precursor to glutathione. This means that a shortage of NAC in the body will limit its ability to make adequate glutathione. It's quite rare that either of the other two components of glutathione, glycine and L-glutamine, will become depleted before cysteine does. It follows that NAC supplementation is the best

radical overload—and as you know from having read this far, that includes most of the diseases that afflict aging people.

The dosage range that has been used in studies ranges from 600 to 3,000 mg. Doses higher than 2,800 mg per day can have pro-oxidant effects in healthy people. To be on the safe side until further research is available, limit NAC use to 2,500 mg per day or less; try 500 mg two to three times per day for starters.

CHAPTER 5

ANTIOXIDANT PHYTOCHEMICALS

Imagine taking a fall walk down a country lane that's lined with tall trees. Picture the leaves, various rich shades of green and gold, red and orange. Visualize fields of tall, pale green grass, dotted with colorful wildflowers. You might even stroll past an apple tree, its branches loaded down with juicy, ripe red apples; a pumpkin vine with its crop nearly ready for Halloween; or a garden filled with leafy green chard and the last few tomatoes of the season.

The reason we're taking this imaginary constitutional is to demonstrate to you that the plant pigments that give all these beauties and delicacies their brilliant colors also happen to be a significant source of their nutrition. Developed by plants over the course of their evolution to protect them against insects, disease, and UV radiation, these pigments nearly all have significant antioxidant activity.

The most abundant class of plant pigments is known as the *carotenoids. Flavonoids* are another type of plant pigment. Both carotenoids and flavonoids are hugely beneficial for human health; many have been found to have benefits that go far beyond their ability to quench free radicals. These pigments turn up in all the foods you probably turned your nose up at as a kid, but they also appear in places where you might not expect them—including chocolate, red wine, and beer!

Plants that are deep green—particularly, the nutritional algaes such as chlorella, spirulina, and

Klamath blue-green algae—contain high concentrations of antioxidant plant pigments called *chlorophyll* and *phycocyanin*. These "superfoods" are known to help protect the body against disease and to delay premature aging, and their antioxidant pigments may be the reason why.

Soy has been a big topic in nutrition circles for years now. It happens to be the richest natural source of *phytochemicals* (plant chemicals) called *genistein* and *daidzein*. Genistein and daidzein are *isoflavones,* substances distantly related to the flavonoids, and their antioxidant activity deserves mention in these pages, too.

Carotenoids: Photosynthetic Nutrients

These fat-soluble nutrients play a critical role in photosynthesis, the metabolic process whereby plants transmute sunshine into energy. Plants make them readily, but animals are—by some evolutionary fluke, perhaps—incapable of synthesizing them. However, most animals can get them from their diet. Carotenoids also create many of the gorgeous colors seen in the animal world, including the pink of flamingo feathers.

In nature, around 700 carotenoids have been discovered, with new varieties continuing to be identified by scientists around the world. They fall into two main categories: the *hydrocarbon carotenoids*, a class that includes beta-carotene, lycopene, and alpha-carotene; and the *xanthophylls,* such as lutein, cryptoxanthin, astaxanthin, and zeaxanthin.

Carotenoids are perfectly biochemically designed to help control free-radical overflow. Without going into too much scientific detail, let's just say that they are uniquely equipped to redistribute their electrons when one is given away to quench a free radical. This gives carotenoids staying power in the midst of the chaotic electron swapping that is constantly going on in the cells.

Carotenoids quench dangerous singlet oxygen radicals and are excellent at terminating free-radical chain reactions.

The carotenoids are best known as precursors to vitamin A—that is, substances that can be transformed into vitamin A, an essential nutrient needed for vision, reproduction, bone growth, maintenance of the skin and the linings of the urinary, respiratory, and intestinal tracts, and support of immunity. About one-third of the vitamin A that the average American adult takes in comes from these carotenoids. Beta-carotene makes the transformation into vitamin A most efficiently.

Carotenoid Research

Research shows that carotenoids protect against cancer, macular degeneration, glaucoma, and heart disease. Animal studies have illustrated that these plant pigments inhibit tumor growth, and that they modulate immunity in ways that help the body suppress the growth of cancers, especially cancers of the breast and prostate. Lycopene, found most abundantly in tomatoes, appears to be a particularly beneficial anticancer nutrient. Lutein and zeaxanthin—xanthophylls found in corn and leafy greens—concentrate in the macula of the retina, protecting the eyes against ultraviolet radiation and other sources of oxidative stress.

A study published in the February 2004 issue of the journal *Arteriosclerosis, Thrombosis, and Vascular Biology* found that antioxidant carotenoids may be protective against early atherosclerosis. Subjects in the Los Angeles Atherosclerosis Study between the ages of forty and sixty were examined twice, once at the beginning of an eighteen-month span and once at the end. They filled out dietary questionnaires and had the thickness of the walls of their carotid artery measured with ultrasound. Fasting blood samples were taken to measure vitamin C, carotenoids, vitamin E, vitamin

A, and cholesterol and inflammatory markers. The results showed that higher levels of lutein, zeaxanthin, beta-cryptoxanthin, and alpha-carotene were associated with decreased progression of carotid wall thickness. Higher levels of lycopene, vitamin C, alpha-carotene, and beta-carotene were associated with lower cholesterol, and higher vitamin C and carotenoid levels were linked with decreased inflammatory markers in the bloodstream (namely, C-reactive protein).

Eat Your Colors!

While supplements of carotenoids are available, so far it seems best to get these nutrients from foods. Foods richest in carotenes are colorful. Filling your plate with at least three different colors at each meal will guarantee that you are getting plenty of these nutrients in your diet. Carrots, yams, pumpkin, peppers, summer squash, tomatoes, corn, leafy greens, cantaloupe, berries, peaches, eggplant, and apples are all carotenoid-rich. Organic produce tends to have more intense color because of higher concentrations of carotenoids and flavonoids.

Some multivitamin and mineral supplements contain lutein, zeaxanthin, and lycopene, and the small boost you'll get from these supplements certainly won't hurt!

Flavonoids

These compounds are, like the carotenoids, found everywhere in nature. *Flavonols, flavones, flavanones, isoflavones, catechins, chalcones,* and *anthocyanidins* are the major classes of flavonoids (also known as bioflavonoids). Within these classes, more than 7,000 different flavonoids have been discovered.

The flavonoids were first discovered by Szent-Gyorgyi, the scientist who discovered vitamin C. He found that the flavonoids often coexisted with vitamin C in foods, and that they had strengthening effects on capillary walls similar to those of vitamin C. Since then, flavonoids have been identified in fruits, vegetables, juices, wine, beer, chocolate, and coffee. According to the website of the Linus Pauling Institute (http://lpi.oregonstate.edu), flavonoids "have been reported to have antiviral, anti-allergic, antiplatelet, anti-inflammatory, antitumor and antioxidant activities" and "epidemiological studies have shown that flavonoid intake is inversely related to mortality from coronary heart disease and to the incidence of heart attacks."

Beer, Chocolate, and Wine— Health Food? Yes!

Researchers at Oregon State University recently discovered a flavanone called *xanthohumol* in hops and beer. When combined with vitamin E, xanthohumol has antioxidant effects superior to those of *quercetin*, another flavonoid that has been the subject of extensive research.

When it was realized that the French, who eat a fattier, higher-cholesterol diet than Americans and have higher blood cholesterol levels, have roughly 2.5 times *lower* probability of developing heart disease, the reason was eventually deduced to be higher intake by the French of flavonoids in red wine, fruits, and vegetables.

Resveratrol, the predominant flavonoid in red wine, has been studied intently since the so-called French paradox was uncovered. At least eight studies demonstrate that drinking one to two glasses of red wine a day protects against heart disease. Red wine drinkers—those who remain moderate—have higher levels of HDL (the "good" cholesterol) and apolipoprotein-A. Red wine flavonoids, which also include rutin and quercetin, powerfully protect LDL against oxidation.

Resveratrol also appears to suppress inflammation. One recent study by researchers at the University of Seville, Spain, found that this red-grape polyphenol suppressed oxidative damage and reduced markers of inflammation in an animal model of inflammatory bowel disease.

A very intriguing new study carried out by Harvard researchers shows that resveratrol may mimic the effects of caloric restriction at the cellular level. Caloric restriction—eating about 30 percent fewer calories than one would naturally consume—has been found to be the most effective way to slow the aging process and ensure a healthy life span.

In one study that linked resveratrol with extension of life span, researchers at MIT used a budding yeast called *Saccharomyces cerevisiae*. It is known that when the caloric intake of *s. cerevisiae* is restricted, the activity of a substance called *Sir2* rises, affecting cellular activity and DNA stability in a way that extends the yeast's life span. When the researchers added resveratrol to a culture of this yeast, it had the same life-extending effect on Sir2.

A study performed at Ninewells Hospital in Scotland showed that flavonoids from dark chocolate decrease *platelet aggregation*, the process that causes blood cells to clump together and clog arteries to the heart or in the brain. Thirty volunteers received 100 grams of either white chocolate, dark chocolate, or milk chocolate. Blood samples taken before the chocolate was eaten, and four hours afterward, showed that the dark chocolate inhibited platelet aggregation by 92 percent. The researchers concluded that flavonoids in the dark chocolate inhibit the COX-1 enzyme that promotes platelet aggregation.

Got Tea? You've Got Flavonoids

Common black and green tea varieties are 25 to 30 percent flavonoids, and these flavonoids have demonstrated heart-protective effects. A forty-year study of Japanese men found that those who drank more green tea had significantly lower cholesterol and triglycerides compared with men who drank less green tea. Tea flavonoids also show huge promise as cancer preventatives.

In a study from Rutgers University, researchers found that drinking black or green tea protects against skin cancer caused by ultraviolet (UV) light and hazardous chemicals. In mice that were given skin cancers through UV or chemical exposure, those that drank black tea had 93 percent fewer tumors than those that drank water. Those that drank green tea had 88 percent fewer tumors than the water drinkers. Decaffeinated tea had slightly less antitumor power.

Here are some of the ways in which tea flavonoids support better health:

- Green tea flavonoids inhibit carcinogen activation—the transformation of relatively harmless substances into carcinogens once they are in the body.

- Tea flavonoids stimulate the action of detoxifying enzymes in the liver, including the p450 detoxification system—an action that helps move carcinogens out of the body before they have a chance to alter DNA activity.

- In cancerous cells, the *tumor suppressor gene* is usually shut off. Green and black tea supplements have been found to turn this gene back on.

- Tea polyphenols are natural inhibitors of *angiogenesis,* the process whereby tumors establish their own circulatory systems.

- Tea also helps to flush excess heavy metals such as mercury, lead, and iron out of the body, which in turn reduces free-radical stress.

Proanthocyanidins: Tongue-Twisting Name for a Quality Antioxidant

While French maritime pine bark is not something you're likely to want to sprinkle on a salad, it does happen to be the source of a flavonoid called *Pycnogenol*. This proanthocyanidin flavonoid is one of about 250 that have been discovered. Grapeseed extract is a source of a similar proanthocyanidin flavonoid.

Hyperbolic claims about, and testimonials to, the incredible healing effects of proanthocyanidins for everything from allergies to heart disease to cancer can be found all over the Internet. When you look at the scientific literature, the picture is clarified: These are simply powerful antioxidant flavonoids, soluble in water. They provide a good complement to other water-soluble antioxidants such as vitamin C and other flavonoids. We also need fat-soluble antioxidants such as vitamin E and the carotenes. It's all about striking a balance.

This is not to say that some of the research into proanthocyanidins isn't promising. Research consistently supports their role in prevention and treatment of circulatory diseases. A recent paper published in *Mutation Research* describes the molecular mechanisms by which a patented proanthocyanidin grapeseed extract (IH636) was shown to protect against heart disease:

- IH636 demonstrated superior antioxidant efficacy compared to vitamins C, E, and beta-carotene [remember that the latter two are fat soluble, which makes this comparison somewhat like comparing apples and oranges];

- IH636 supplementation improved functional assessments of heart function, including improved pumping strength, decreased size of heart attack, decreased incidence of dangerous heartbeat irregularities, and decreased reactive oxygen species (free radical) formation in the heart;

- Supplementation of 50 milligrams (mg) of IH636 per kilogram (kg) of body weight reduced formation of foam cells—an early marker of atherosclerosis—by 49 percent, while 100 mg/kg reduced foam-cell formation by 63 percent.

Grapeseed extract (GSE) has also been found to significantly decrease LDL oxidation. In one study, smokers who used grapeseed extract supplements had 20 percent lower measurements of LDL oxidation than smokers who did not. Other measurements showed that the LDL of the smokers who used GSE supplements was better able, by 15 percent, to resist oxidative stress.

In the animal model of diabetes, researchers cause the disease by giving rats a poison called streptozotocin; soon after it is given, their blood glucose levels rise and free-radical production in their livers rises. A group of Kenyan researchers gave a group of their diabetic rats a Pycnogenol supplement, and found that it restored to normal the activity of an endogenous antioxidant called *catalase* in their livers. They also found that diabetic rats treated with Pycnogenol had significant elevations in levels of reduced glutathione and in glutathione-associated enzyme function.

In a study by Irish researchers, Pycnogenol was found to inhibit the release of the inflammatory chemical *histamine*—the stuff that causes itchy, runny noses and eyes during allergy season—from mast cells, the immune cells that make it.

Bioflavonoids: A Good Reason to Eat Citrus

Many of the bioflavonoids found in citrus fruits seem to have redundant benefits. For example, most of them offer protection against cancer. And, the research shows, they do so through a variety of biological mechanisms.

Citrus bioflavonoids protect against ischemia/reperfusion injury in animal models, as well, most likely due to their antioxidant actions.

Here's a sampling of the research on citrus flavonoids:

- *Hesperidin,* abundant in oranges and lemons, was found in an animal study to reduce cancerous and precancerous tongue lesions by 62 percent. Other research showed that supplementing with hesperidin enhanced bone resorption of calcium, phosphorus, and zinc, and prevented bone loss in an animal model of menopause. Further studies suggest that it could help reduce high blood pressure.

- *Naringin,* found in grapefruit, reduced DNA damage from radiation in one study of bone marrow cells; the risk of developing leukemia decreased as a result. *Naringenin,* a closely related compound, has been found to inhibit the growth of colon cancer cells in test tube studies.

- *Limonene* is abundant in lemons and oranges. It has been used in high doses to slow the growth of breast tumors, with some success. This flavonoid also appears to help forestall the growth of colon and pancreatic cancers. A Chinese study illustrated that limonene also induces apoptosis (cell death) in stomach cancer cells.

- *Nobiletin* is found in flat lemon, a fruit popular in Japan. This flavonoid has been found to inhibit the production of pro-inflammatory biochemicals, notably *prostaglandin E2.* Animal studies suggest that nobiletin could be an effective treatment for osteoarthritis, and that it inhibits the metastasis (spread) of stomach cancers.

- *Diosmin,* found in lemons and oranges, has been found to reduce oral tumors and pre-cancerous cell changes in an animal model of smoking and tobacco chewing. Along with hes-peridin, it has been found to protect against capillary fragility caused by allergic reactions.

Eating citrus fruits is the best way to get healthy helpings of these bioflavonoids. Juices don't pack the same nutrient punch as the pulp and rind. Try recipes that call for citrus zest—grated rind—in addition to eating whole fruit. Of course, lemons and limes are not so good for eating, so use their zest in sauces for chicken and fish. (Organic citrus is the best way to go here, because nonorganic citrus is sprayed with all kinds of chemicals.)

If you take prescription medication, be aware that grapefruit is probably not your best choice. It contains furanocoumarins and P-glycoprotein, which enhance the absorption of many drugs and can cause an overdose. Stick with oranges, lemon, and lime.

You can take a bioflavonoid supplement; choose a mixed supplement that delivers 700–1,500 milligrams per day.

Heart-Protective Soy Isoflavones

Isoflavones are a type of flavonoid found only in soybeans and in some herbs (dong quai, black cohosh, licorice, and red clover). Several studies have demonstrated that isoflavones have significant antioxidant capability. Other research shows that they can modulate risk of heart attack by improving the ability of arteries to relax and by reducing arterial inflammation.

Soy isoflavones, more than any other flavonoid, act like weak estrogens in the body. (Other flavonoids have this effect as well but to a lesser extent.) Their estrogenic effects are milder than those of estrogens made in the ovaries, and much weaker than those of environmental estrogens, or *xenoestrogens*—synthetic chemical versions of estrogens that are carcinogenic because of their high-powered estrogenic activity.

The most studied of the isoflavones are *genistein* and *daidzein*. Their potential uses range from natural hormone replacement for menopause symptoms, for prevention of osteoporosis, and for prevention of colon cancer. University of Michigan researchers found that genistein reduced precancerous colon polyp occurrence by 40 percent in rats that were genetically susceptible to colon cancer.

Research into genistein's usefulness as a breast cancer preventative has been somewhat controversial. Some studies suggest that concentrated soy isoflavones encourage breast cancer growth, while others suggest that they block it or slow it down. To be on the safe side, women who have been diagnosed with breast cancer should avoid genistein supplements. (They can eat soy foods without worry.) Research indicates that women who eat soy in their younger years—during adolescence—are most likely to gain anti–breast cancer benefits from that soy later on.

With what is known today, the best way to add more genistein and daidzein to your life is by eating soy foods. Tofu, tempeh, miso, soy milk, soy protein powder-based smoothies, and soy burgers are all good ways to add soy to your diet. Try to eat soy once a day.

Chlorophyll and Phycocyanin: Deepest Green Plant Pigments

Chlorophyll and phycocyanin are, respectively, the green and blue pigments that give green plants and blue-green algae their beautiful colors. Chlorophyll enables plants to make energy from sunshine. Both compounds are being studied intensively in labs across the world because of their promise as anticancer agents.

Phycocyanin has strong antioxidant and free-radical-scavenging effects. It acts as a COX-2 inhibitor, decreasing the production of inflammatory prostaglandins that have been linked with both heart disease and cancer. There have been reports of induction of apoptosis (cancer cell death) by drugs that inhibit COX-2.

Blue-green plant pigments appear to shield us against cancer through several mechanisms. Japanese researchers analyzed blood cells for anticancer interferon activity before and after a dose of blue-green algae. As expected, their production of interferon gamma rose, as did other functions of their natural killer (NK) cells. Inhibitory effects on cultured liver cancer cells have been found with blue-green algae supplements.

Scientists in India found that phycocyanin enhanced phase II liver detoxification, which is the most important for ridding the body of carcinogens. They also found increases in antioxidant enzymes and the antioxidant glutathione, and decreases in lipid peroxidation. When the mice given phycocyanin were challenged with carcinogens, they developed smaller tumors, with fewer tumors overall than mice that did not get phycocyanin.

According to studies from the Linus Pauling Institute at Oregon State University, chlorophyllin (a derivative of chlorophyll) decreases the proliferation of breast and colon cancer cells. In one study of human colon cancer cells, chlorophyllin caused growth arrest within twenty-four hours and apoptosis soon after, and appeared to defend against cancer at both the initiation and growth stages.

Aflatoxin B_1, a potent liver toxin, is the cause of most cases of liver cancer worldwide. Studies performed with chlorophyll suggest that it will turn out to be our best protection against liver cancer in populations that cannot avoid having it in their diets.

Blue-green algae has been found to help reverse the growth of lesions in the mouth that are the predecessors of oral cancer. Rinsing the mouth with a solution of spirulina can slow the growth of oral cancer.

CHAPTER 6

HERBAL ANTIOXIDANTS

The tradition of herbal medicine extends back as far as human history. If the present-day behavior of many animal species is any indication, it likely goes back a lot farther.

Monkeys, lemurs, bears, and many other creatures have been observed in the wild medicating themselves with specific plants. For example, chimpanzees with diarrhea will range far and wide to find a plant called *Vernonia amygdalina*. They chew pulp from the center of the plant, and it cures them. African people who live nearby make a decoction of the same plant to treat intestinal parasites. Madagascar lemurs eat plants rich in tannins in the weeks before giving birth; in small doses, these otherwise toxic tannins have been found to support milk production and protect against miscarriage. Bears make an herbal paste that repels insects, which they smear on their own fur.

Scientists who learn about herbal medicine from animal self-medication are practicing a new science called *zoopharmacognosy*. What we learn from them can add to our long human tradition of herbal medicine—which, today, is gaining huge ground due to science's ability to analyze the so-called active constituents of plant medicines. Many of these active constituents, it turns out, have significant antioxidant activity. The best-understood of the antioxidant herbs are milk thistle, ginkgo biloba, curcumin, and garlic.

Milk Thistle (*Silybum Marianum*): Liver Supporter, Glutathione Booster

Traditional uses for milk thistle (*Silybum marianum*) have included treatment of varicose veins, menstrual problems, depression, and low breast-milk production. By far its most valuable use, however, is as a liver supporter.

The liver works constantly, day in and day out, to remove toxic substances from the blood that circulate in the body. Each of its two lobes uses complex enzymatic processes to neutralize toxins and direct them out of the body through the intestinal or urinary tracts. Drugs, used-up hormones and immune cells, man-made chemicals, excess heavy metals, and toxins naturally found in food, all have to be detoxified by the liver in order to be eliminated safely. Inadequate liver function leads to a rapid buildup of toxins in this organ, damaging it and causing toxins to leak out into the general circulation.

Liver detoxification makes a great number of free radicals. This is why the liver contains such high concentrations of endogenous antioxidants, particularly glutathione.

In the modern world, where pollutants and prescription drugs are common aspects of life, the liver has its work cut out for it. Milk thistle has been used to treat liver disorders, including cirrhosis and hepatitis, since Roman times. Modern research is showing that its active constituent, the flavonoid *silymarin*, has remarkable antioxidant power that centers in the tissues of the liver.

Uses for Milk Thistle

Milk thistle is the antidote to death cap mushroom (*Amanita phalloides*) poisoning. When the mushroom is eaten, it promptly kills off 30 to 40 percent of the cells of the liver by depleting them of glutathione. Taking large doses of milk thistle can be lifesaving if you've swallowed the wrong kind of mushroom.

Milk thistle protects the liver against man-made poisons, including carbon tetrachloride (an industrial solvent used for dry cleaning), thioacetamide (a man-made chemical that causes cirrhosis), and heavy metals. It is an effective treatment for liver poisoning from acetaminophen (Tylenol) overdose.

Milk thistle efficiently neutralizes free radicals in the liver, in part by raising levels of glutathione peroxidase and superoxide dismutase (another antioxidant enzyme) in liver cells. Milk thistle also inhibits the production of biochemicals that accelerate excessive inflammation in the liver—inflammation that goes hand in hand with excessive free-radical production.

Milk thistle also stimulates the growth of new liver cells. It is so powerful in this regard that it literally regenerates liver tissues. Studies suggest that phytochemicals from milk thistle protect liver cells against DNA damage, stabilize *mast cells* (immune cells that drive the inflammatory process), and bind to excess iron so that it can be removed from the body.

Milk thistle may also be useful therapy for diabetes. In a study by Chinese researchers, fourteen patients with type 2 diabetes took milk thistle for four weeks. Their red blood cell sorbitol levels—a measurement of high blood sugar—dropped 50 percent, and the speed of their nerve impulses improved.

Psoriasis, an inflammatory skin condition, has also been controlled with milk thistle supplementation. This may be due to improved liver detoxification, which would rid the body of toxins to which the skin reacts; or, it may be due to milk thistle's anti-inflammatory effects.

Gallstones are the reason for about 300,000 gallbladder removal surgeries per year in the United States. These stones are caused by thickened bile, which can be thinned with milk thistle. Some research indicates that flavonoids from milk thistle help the kidneys to fulfill their role in the detoxification process. Milk thistle has demonstrated the ability to slow the growth of human breast, prostate, and cervical cancer cells in test-tube studies.

If you would like to try taking milk thistle, choose a standardized extract (70 to 80 percent silymarin) totaling 70 to 210 milligrams. Take this dose three times daily. Higher doses can be beneficial for those with liver disease; consult an herbalist or naturopath if you would like to try high-dose milk thistle to help heal your liver.

Ginkgo Biloba: Brain-Health Promoter and Anticancer Agent

The ginkgo trees alive today are exactly like those that lived during the time of the dinosaurs. Fossils of these hardy trees date back to 270 million years ago.

In Hiroshima, about a kilometer from the epicenter of the detonation of the nuclear bomb at the end of World War II, there is a ginkgo tree that survived the blast. In fact, it is said to have budded soon after the blast without major deformations, although the temple it was planted in front of was completely destroyed. Three other such trees survive in Japan; one still has scorch marks on its trunk from the explosion.

A plant that has survived for this long, that can endure the blast of a thermonuclear bomb, must have something to teach us. Turns out that it does: ginkgo happens to be one of the most valuable herbal medicines around. It has particular promise for slowing the progression of Alzheimer's disease (AD). Germany recently approved it as a treatment for this progressive form of dementia.

Ginkgo phytochemicals—specifically, terpenoids and flavonoids—enhance blood flow in the brain and throughout the body. They have pronounced antioxidant and anti-inflammatory actions; test-tube studies have illustrated that ginkgo extracts enhance cellular redox (reduction) state and raise levels of *nitric oxide*, a naturally occurring chemical that opens up blood vessels. Multiple trials have shown that ginkgo therapy can slow the deterioration of memory and thinking ability in people with AD.

The best known of these studies was published in the *Journal of the American Medical Association* in 1997. Its authors, LeBars et al., stated that ginkgo extract is "safe and appears capable of stabilizing and, in a substantial number of cases, improving the cognitive performance and the social function of demented patients for six months to one year." These effects were as dramatic as those seen with commonly prescribed AD medications such as tacrine and Aricept.

It is likely that this effect of ginkgo is due to a combination of its ability to protect against oxidation, particularly lipid peroxidation, and the anticlotting and anti-inflammatory effects of its terpenoids. More research is underway, some of it government funded.

Terpenoids
Naturally occurring chemicals; many varieties are found in plants and give them their characteristic scents and flavors.

Ginkgo also happens to have some impressive anticancer effects. Aside from preventing DNA oxidation, it also inhibits angiogenesis (the growth of blood vessels to feed tumors) and appears to have some gene-regulatory actions. One study found a decrease in proliferation of a highly aggressive human breast cancer strain when ginkgo extract was used; another study of ginkgo illustrated that human bladder cancer cells underwent changes that made them less dangerous. Human studies show that ginkgo extracts inhibit the precancerous changes induced by ultraviolet and other types of radiation. The authors of a 2003 review in *Fundamentals of Clinical Pharmacology*, Defeudis, et al., summarize, ". . . [the] flavonoid and terpenoid constituents of Ginkgo extracts may act in a complementary manner to inhibit several carcinogenesis-related processes." Research is still in its early stages, but so far it's pretty promising.

The proper dose of ginkgo biloba extract will depend upon its standardization. Stick with the dosage recommended on the packaging of the extract you choose.

Curcumin *(Curcuma Longa)*: Multifaceted Cancer Fighter

Turmeric (*Curcuma longa*), a bright yellow-orange spice that belongs to the ginger family, has been used as a culinary spice and a medicinal herb for thousands of years. Today, it is most commonly used as a flavoring in Indian and other Asian foods. Ayurvedic and Chinese traditional medical practitioners use curcumin—a derivative of turmeric—in their herbal medicines. Mainstream science has caught wind of the amazing health-promoting effects of curcumin, and studies of its various salutary effects are now in progress all over the world. A large body of research already indicates that curcumin may well be our most powerful natural ally in the fight against cancer.

Test-tube studies show that curcumin has respectable antioxidant punch, but its ability to counter the effects of free radicals on fats and DNA is only a small part of its anticancer strategy. Research has uncovered several additional ways in which curcumin helps to prevent cancer:

- Curcumin fits through a cellular "doorway" that also allows estrogen-mimicking xenobiotics into cells. The phytochemical fills the doorway, preventing carcinogenic xenoestrogens from entering. In one test-tube study, the growth of human breast cancer cells enhanced by 17-beta estradiol—the strongest natural estrogen—was blocked 98 percent; the growth of cancer cells to which the xenobiotic DDT was added slowed by 75 percent when curcumin was also added; and the effect of a combination of the toxic chemicals chlordane and endosulfane, which as a rule greatly enhance breast cancer growth, was inhibited 90 percent with curcumin. (The addition of genistein as well as curcumin completely stopped the cancerous cells from growing!)

- Curcumin also blocks other, non-estrogenic chemicals that cause cancer, including diethylnitrosamine and dioxins.

- Curcumin is a natural *kinase inhibitor,* which means that it cuts off communications within cancer cells. This inhibits their growth. Drug companies are presently trying to formulate synthetic kinase inhibitors for use as cancer drugs.

- Curcumin blocks the activity of cancer growth factors such as NF-kappa B, certain cytokines, protein kinase C, and interleukin-8.

- Curcumin is a natural inhibitor of the inflammation-causing COX enzymes; people who take synthetic COX-inhibitor drugs have been found to have a significantly reduced risk of some cancers.

- In a test-tube study, curcumin prevented virtually all DNA damage in bacteria that were exposed to lethal doses of radiation.

- Curcumin encourages apoptosis in cancerous cells, but not in healthy ones.

- Curcumin interrupts the cycle of cancer cells at a particular stage of growth. One study found that combining curcumin with ECGC, the major flavonoid in green tea, interrupted the cancer cell cycle at two separate stages.

- A study by Indian researchers found that curcumin protects liver glutathione concentrations and supports *DNA methylation*.

- Meat cooked over an open flame forms carcinogenic chemicals. A meat marinade made with turmeric was shown to reduce the formation of these chemicals.

DNA Methylation
A biochemical process that constantly goes on within the cells, keeping tumor-suppressing genes turned on and tumor-promoting genes turned off.

As if these cancer-preventing effects weren't enough to recommend it, curcumin also has proven benefits for immunity (enhancement of antibody production and immune system activity), wound healing (when topically applied), and heart health (it reduces blood lipids and prevents LDL oxidation). It is both bactericidal and antiprotozoal.

If you've never been a big eater of curries, now may be the time to start trying them. You can also take supplemental curcumin; follow the dosage instructions on the label, which will vary depending upon the concentration of active constituents in the extract. If you have cancer and wish to try higher doses, consult with your oncologist and a naturopath to make sure you are using them safely.

Garlic: The Fragrant Healer

Another herb with a long history of both culinary and medicinal use, garlic often inspires either love or hate. Some will eat it in or on virtually everything, while others avoid it because they don't like the taste or are concerned that it will cause them to have a less-than-pleasant odor. One thing's for sure: the scientifically proven health benefits of garlic are nothing to sniff at.

Garlic has cholesterol- and triglyceride-lowering, anticlotting, antibacterial, and antitumor effects. And, of course, its main constituents—sulfur-containing phytochemicals such as S-allylcysteine, S-allylmercapto-L-cysteine, and other allyl sulfides—do battle with free radicals with the best of the antioxidants.

Organosulfur compounds are found in onions, garlic, shallots, scallions, and chives. Population studies have shown repeatedly that cancer incidence is lowest where the consumption of organosulfur-rich foods is greatest. Animal and test-tube studies have shown that organosulfur compounds induce apoptosis in skin tumors, and that they protect against liver cancer caused by aflatoxin. Further research indicates that diallyl sulfide (another of the organosulfur compounds) inhibits the growth of human breast cancer cells. Most evidence as to why garlic has such potent anticancer effects points to the ability of organosulfur compounds to affect the action of drug metabolism enzymes, heighten antioxidant activity, and directly inhibit the growth of tumors.

One study, by Dr. T. Abdullah of the Akbar Clinic and Research Institute in Panama, Florida, illustrates how garlic boosts anticancer immune function. The subjects ate raw garlic or Kyolic (an aged garlic extract), then had blood drawn, as did a control group who ate no garlic. The blood samples were evaluated for natural killer cell function when mixed in a lab dish with cancer cells. Natural killer cells from the garlic eaters destroyed 140 to 160 percent more cancer cells than the blood from non-garlic eaters.

In six of ten studies, garlic extracts rich in allicin (you guessed it, also an organosulfur compound) lowered total blood cholesterol by an average of 24.8 milligrams per deciliter (mg/dL), LDL by an average of 15.3 mg/dL, and triglycerides 38 mg/dL—all significant enough to have an effect on heart disease risk. The anticlotting effects of garlic extract help prevent clogged blood vessels in the heart, legs, and brain.

The U.S. Department of Agriculture's Human Nutrition Center in Beltsville, Maryland, has done research that demonstrates an antidiabetic effect of garlic. Their research showed decreases in blood sugar and improvements in insulin activity with garlic.

Aged garlic extracts appear to be the best way to reap the benefits of garlic without constantly smelling like an Italian kitchen. Cook with garlic whenever you can, though; it provides a delicious complement to most meats and vegetables. If everyone in your household eats it, no one will complain about garlic breath later on!

CONCLUSION

Now that you've almost completed your whirlwind tour through the world of antioxidant nutrition, you may have more questions than answers. You may have been impressed by the promise of these nutrients for the promotion of excellent health, but you may also wonder how to add them all to your supplement program without breaking the bank or having to take ten pills at every meal.

Simplicity and balance are of the essence when it comes to nutrient supplementation. While the research into antioxidants is hugely promising, it isn't far enough along to guarantee the safety of using high doses of several antioxidants for long periods. Seek out a multivitamin and mineral supplement that is formulated with as many of the antioxidants as possible, in balanced amounts; eat a diet filled with antioxidant-rich fruits, vegetables, herbs, and spices; and use higher doses of antioxidants for disease treatment sparingly and with the guidance of a nutrition expert or naturopath.

There is no known health risk, however, in supplementing with all of the nutrients described in these pages, all at the same time, as long as you keep within the moderate dosages that are recommended on the packaging. Don't think that doing so exempts you from having to eat a good diet, though. Much of the research on antioxidant benefits is based on taking them in through nutritious foods. Even those studies that indicate benefits from supplements are often skewed by the fact that people who use nutrient supplements tend to be more health conscious in general and eat better diets.

Maintain balance in your antioxidant supplementation. Don't use high doses of one without balance from others. Use the knowledge you have gained in these pages to create a program that works for you. You'll feel better, look better, and you'll have a better chance of living longer and remaining free of chronic diseases such as heart disease, diabetes, and Alzheimer's disease.

Enjoy!

SELECTED REFERENCES

Aggarwal BB, Kumar A, Bharti AC. "Anticancer potential of curcumin: preclinical and clinical studies." *Anticancer Res.* 2003 Jan/Feb;23(1A):363–398.

Ames BN. "A role for supplements in optimizing health: the metabolic tune-up." *Archives of Biochemistry and Biophysics.* 2004 Mar 1;423(1):227–234.

Antony S, et al. "Immunomodulatory activity of curcumin." *Immunol Invest.* 1999;28:291–303.

Bagchi D, et al. "Molecular mechanisms of cardioprotection by a novel grapeseed proanthocyanidin extract." *Mutation Research.* 2003 Feb/Mar; 523–24: 87–97.

Bosisio E, et al. "Effect of the flavanolignans of *Silybum marianum L.* on lipid peroxidation in rat liver microsomes and freshly isolated hepatocytes." *Pharmacol Res.* 1992;25:147–154.

Bouskela E, Cyrino FZ, Lerond L. "Effects of oral administration of different doses of purified micronized flavonoid fraction on microvascular reactivity after ischaemia/reperfusion in the hamster cheek pouch." *Br J Pharmacol.* 1997 Dec;122(8):1611–6.

Campos R, et al. "Silybin dihemisuccinate protects against glutathione depletion and lipid peroxidation induced by acetaminophen on rat liver." *Planta Med.* 1989;55:417–419.

Chiba H, et al. "Hesperidin, a citrus flavonoid, inhibits bone loss and decreases serum and hepatic lipids in ovariectomized mice." *J Nutr.* 2003 Jun;133(6):1892–1897.

Crestanello JA, et al. "Effect of coenzyme Q_{10} supplementation on mitochondrial function after myocardial ischemia reperfusion." *J Surg Res.* 2002 Feb;102(2):221–228.

Crowell PL, Siar Ayoubi A, Burke YD. "Antitumorigenic effects of limonene and perillyl alcohol against pancreatic and breast cancer." *Adv Exp Med Biol.* 1996; 401:131–136.

De Flora S, Grassi C, Carati L. "Attenuation of influenza-like symptomatology and improvement of cell-mediated immunity with long-term N-acetylcysteine treatment." *Eur Resp J.* 1997;10:1535–1541.

De La Puerta R, Martinez E, Bravo L. "Effect of silymarin on different acute inflammation models and on leukocyte migration." *J Pharm Pharmacol.* 1996;48: 968–970.

DeFeudis FV, Papadopoulos V, Prien K. "Ginkgo biloba extracts and cancer: a research area in its infancy." *Fundam Clin Pharmacol.* 2003 Aug;17(4):405–417.

Dehmlow C, et al. "Scavenging of reactive oxygen species and inhibition of arachidonic acid metabolism by silibinin in human cells." *Life Sci.* 1996;58: 1591–1600.

Desplaces A, et al. The effects of silymarin on experimental phalloidine poisoning." *Arzneimittelforschung.* 1975;25:89–96.

Elattar TM, et al. "The inhibitory effect of curcumin, genistein, quercetin and cisplatin on the growth of oral cancer cells in vitro." *Anticancer Res.* 2000;20(3A): 1733–1738.

Ferenci P, et al. "Randomized controlled trial of silymarin treatment in patients with cirrhosis of the liver." *J Hepatol.* 1989;9:105–113.

Fiebrich F, Koch H. "Silymarin, an inhibitor of lipoxygenase." *Experentia.* 1979;35:150–152.

Folkers K, Sartori M, Baker L, Richardson P. "Observations of significant reductions of arrhythmias in treatment with coenzyme Q_{10} of patients having cardiovascular disease." *IRCS Medical Science.* 1982;10: 348–349.

Frydoonfar HR, McGrath DR, Spiegelman AD. "The variable effect of proliferation of a colon cancer cell line by the citrus fruit flavonoid naringenin." *Colorectal Dis.* 2003 Mar;5(2):149–152.

"Glutathione/reduced GSH: technical monograph." *Alt Med Rev.* 2001 Dec;6(6).

Halim AB, et al. "Biochemical effect of antioxidants on lipids and liver function in experimentally-induced liver damage." *Ann Clin Biochem.* 1997;34:656–663.

Herzenberg LA, de Rosa SC, Dubs JG, et al. "Glutathione deficiency is associated with impaired survival in HIV disease." *Proc Natl Acad Sci USA.* 1997;94: 1967–1972.

Hikino H, et al. "Antihepatotoxic actions of flavonolignans from *Silybum marianum* fruits." *Planta Medica.* 1984;50:248–250.

Hock C, et al. "Increased blood mercury levels in patients with Alzheimer's disease." *Neural Transm.* 1998;105(1):59–68.

Jagetia CG, Venkatesha VA, Reddy TK. "Naringin, a citrus flavonone, protects against radiation-induced chromosome damage in mouse bone marrow." *Mutagenesis.* 2003 Jul;18(4):337–43.

Jobin C, et al. "Curcumin blocks cytokine-mediated NF-kappa B activation and proinflammatory gene expression by inhibiting inhibitory factor I-kappa B kinase activity." *J Immunol.* 163:3474–83.

Kawamori T, et al. "Chemopreventive effect of curcumin, a naturally occurring anti-inflammatory agent, during the promotion/progression stages of colon cancer." *Cancer Res.* 1999;59:597–601.

Kreeman V, et al. "Silymarin inhibits the development of diet-induced hypercholesterolemia in rats." *Planta Med.* 1998;64:138–142.

Kuklinski B, Weissenbacher E, Fahnrich A. "Coenzyme Q_{10} and antioxidants in acute myocardial infarction." *Mol Aspects Med.* 1994;15Suppl:S143–S147.

Langsjoen PH. "Effective and safe therapy with coenzyme Q_{10} for cardiomyopathy. *Klinische Wochenschrift.* 1988;66:583–590.

Lavy A, et al. *Ann Nutr Metab.* 1994 Sept/Oct; 38: 287–294.

LeBars, et al. "A placebo-controlled, double-blind, randomized trial of an extract of ginkgo biloba for dementia." *JAMA.* 1997;278(16):1327–1332.

Lertratanangkoon K, et al. "Inhibition of glutathione synthesis with proppargylglycine enhances N-acetyl-methionine protection and methylation in bromo-benzene-treated Syrian hamsters." *J Nutr.* 1999;129: 649–656.

Lin N, et al. "Novel anti-inflammatory actions of nobiletin, a citrus polymethoxy flavonoid, on human synovial fibroblasts and mouse macrophages." *Biochem Pharmacol.* 2003 Jun 15;65(12):2065–2071.

Lockwood, K. "Partial and complete regression of breast cancer in patients in relation to dosage of co-enzyme Q_{10}." *Biochemical and Biophysical Research Communications.* 1994 Mar 30;199:1504–1508.

Lu XG, et al. "D-limonene induces apoptosis of gastric cancer cells." *Zhonggua Zhong Liu Za Zhi.* 2003 Jul; 25(4):325–327.

Luper S. "A review of plants used in the treatment of liver disease: part 1." *Altern Med Rev.* 1998;4:410–421.

Manthey JA. "Biological properties of flavonoids pertaining to inflammation." *Microcirculation.* 2000;7(6 Pt 2):S29–S34.

Maritim A, et al. "Effects of Pycnogenol treatment on oxidative stress in streptozotocin-induced diabetic rats." *Biochem Mol Toxicol.* 2003;17(3):193–199.

Martin AR, et al. "Resveratrol, a polyphenol found in grapes, suppresses oxidative damage and stimulates apoptosis during early colonic inflammation in rats." *Biochem Pharmacol.* 2004 Apr 1;67(7):1399–1410.

Munch G, et al. "Anti-AGEing defences against Alzheimer disease." *Biochem Soc Trans.* 2003 Dec;31 (Pt 6):1297.

Oyama, et al. "Ginkgo biloba extract protects brain neurons against oxidative stress induced by hydrogen peroxide." *Brain Research.* 1996;712:349–352.

"Resveratrol may increase lifespan." *Natural Products Industry Insider.* 2003 Sept 10:16. Study published online at www.nature.com/ on August 24, 2003.

Sierpina VS, Wollschlaeger, Blumenthal M. "Ginkgo biloba." *Am Fam Physician.* 2003 Sep 1;68(5):923–926.

Simon J, et al. "Relation of serum ascorbic acid to mortality among U.S. adults." *J Am Coll Nutr.* 2001;20(3).

Steinberg FM, et al. "Soy protein with isoflavones has favorable effects on endothelial function that are independent of lipid and antioxidant effects in healthy postmenopausal women." *Am J Clin Nutr.* 2003 Jul; 78(1):123–130.

Tanaka T, et al. "Chemoprevention of 4-nitroquinoline 1-oxide-induced oral carcinogenesis in rats by flavonoids diosmin and hesperidin, each alone and in combination." *Cancer Res.* 1997 Jan 15;57(2):246–252.

Verma SP, et al. "Curcumin and genistein, plant natural products, show synergistic inhibitory effects on the growth of human breast cancer MCF-7 cells induced by estrogenic pesticides." *Biochem Biphy Res Comm.* 1997;233:692–696.

Verma SP, et al. "The inhibition of the estrogenic effects of pesticides and environmental chemicals by curcumin and isoflavonoids." *Environ Health Perspect.* 1998;106:807–812.

Witting PL, et al. "Anti-atherogenic effect of coenzyme Q_{10} in alipoprotein E gene knockout mice." *Free Radic Biol Med.* 2000;29(3–4):295–305.

Yen GC, Lai HH. "Inhibition of reactive nitrogen species effects in vitro and in vivo by isoflavones and soy-based food extracts." *J Agric Food Chem.* 2003 Dec 31;51(27):7892–7900.

OTHER BOOKS
AND RESOURCES

GreatLife Magazine

Consumer magazine with articles on vitamins, minerals, herbs, and foods.

Available for free at many health and natural food stores.

Let's Live Magazine

Consumer magazine with emphasis on the health benefits of vitamins, minerals, and herbs.

Customer service:

1-800-676-4333

P.O. Box 74908

Los Angeles, CA 90004

Subscriptions: 12 issues per year, $19.95 in the U.S.; $31.95 outside the U.S.

Physical Magazine

Magazine oriented to body builders and other serious athletes.

Customer service:

1-800-676-4333

P.O. Box 74908

Los Angeles, CA 90004

Subscriptions: 12 issues per year, $19.95 in the U.S.; $31.95 outside the U.S.

The Nutrition Reporter™ newsletter

Monthly newsletter that summarizes recent medical research on vitamins, minerals, and herbs.

Customer service:

P.O. Box 30246

Tucson, AZ 85751-0246

e-mail: jack@thenutritionreporter.com

www.nutritionreporter.com

Subscriptions: 12 issues per year, $26 in the U.S.; $32 U.S. or $48 CNC for Canada; $38 for other countries.

INDEX

Printed in the USA
CPSIA information can be obtained
at www.ICGtesting.com
JSHW012007140824
68134JS00004B/48